TINY MEDICINE

"*Tiny Medicine* offers a rare, behind-the-scenes, look into the life and work of one of our nation's leading neonatologists, Dr. Chris DeRienzo. Full of compelling stories, humor, and raw emotional vulnerability, DeRienzo takes us on a journey through the joys and tragedies of caring for the smallest patients, often in life or death situations. This is a must read for anyone interested in peeking behind the curtain of modern healthcare into the real world of tiny medicine."
–Nate Klemp, PhD, co-founder of LIFE XT and co-author of the *New York Times* Bestseller *Start Here: Master The Lifelong Habit of Wellbeing*

"With one glance, Dr. DeRienzo creates a human connection with his patients and reminds us that we need technologies that build trust, value the sacred relationship between a doctor and a patient, and restore the patient voice and narrative back to healthcare. He gives the reader hope that healthcare can be healed."
–Dr. Bridget Duffy, MD, CMO of Vocera Communications, Inc.

TINY MEDICINE

ONE DOCTOR'S BIGGEST LESSONS FROM HIS SMALLEST PATIENTS

———

DR. CHRIS DERIENZO

BIG EYE BOOKS

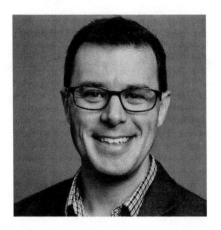

Dr. Chris DeRienzo is a dedicated husband, proud father, mediocre triathlete, and a physician committed to improving America's health and returning humanity to the practice of medicine. Recognized by *Modern Healthcare* as one of 15 "Up and Comers" Under 40, Chris currently serves as Chief Medical Officer for Cardinal Analytx and sees his patients in the Mission Children's NICU follow-up clinic. A frequent keynote speaker on the intersection of humanity and technology in healthcare, he advises both state and national governments and companies from early-stage ventures to the Fortune 500 on issues related to healthcare quality, safety, and analytics. He's also a sucker for bucket list races, a frequent early-morning Zwift rider, and can quote *The West Wing's* "Two Cathedrals" episode line-for-line… including the Latin swearing. Chris lives with his family and their two remarkably energetic dogs in Asheville, NC.

Tiny Medicine:
One Doctor's Biggest Lessons from His Smallest Patients

Big Eye Books
Athens, GA

www.bigeyebooks.com

ISBN: 978-1-7337335-0-2
eISBN: 978-1-7337335-1-9

Printed in the United States of America

1 2 3 4 5 6 7 8 9 10

Jacket design: Boo Gilder
Cover illustration: Kaylyn Venuto

To Munchkin, Bean, and Chief, for making me a better doctor and a better person by continuously making me become a better father.

CONTENTS

Foreword

I first met Dr. Chris DeRienzo through his mentor, Dr. Ron Paulus, at Mission Health while he served as Mission's Chief Quality Officer. As a fierce advocate for patient quality and safety, Chris was an early supporter of the LIFE Cross Training program that helps professionals build resilience, attain optimal wellbeing, and achieve peak personal performance. Chris' passion for the subject stood out—and his commitment to helping his colleagues inspired me and those around him. I grew to know Chris as a gentle, kind person, with a giant caring heart and strong focus on values. Now, after reading *Tiny Medicine*, I know him both as a humble leader "standing tall" on the deck steering into incredible adversity and challenges and as a driven competitor, participating in an Ironman Triathlon and sprinting down hospital hallways to save the lives of the most vulnerable among us.

Tiny Medicine takes us on a journey inside the inner operations of the U.S. healthcare industry. Employing 1 in 5 people in our country, healthcare is now the nation's largest industry, having surpassed retail and manufacturing employment in early 2018. It also could easily be considered our country's most vital and important industry. Yet, despite this behemoth scale, most of us have very little insight into what it truly is like to live and work inside this world where life-and-death decisions are literally made moment by moment. Chris' tale gives a glimpse inside this veiled world in which physicians are put through grueling training programs and routinely asked to engage in emotionally draining work that leaves them frazzled and vulnerable to exhaustion, dissatisfaction, and burnout.

Tiny Medicine is a timely book. Despite the giant economic scale of the healthcare industry, our healthcare system is a human one by its very nature. For the consumers of its product, it's the very humanity of this system that matters. In the account that follows, Dr. Chris DeRienzo, a neonatologist and pediatrician, an Ironman, a triathlete, a father, a sought-after international speaker and community volunteer, offers us a humble, authentic, and unassuming view into his experiences as a physician. Without any self-consciousness or trace of ego, Chris shares his personal account of his taxingly ambitious journey through today's healthcare system, from his initial yearnings to practice medicine to his learning to "stand tall on the deck" as a lead Fellow at Duke's neonatal intensive care unit (NICU). As we travel along the journey with him, he reveals with a disarming candor the highs and lows of his experience—including clinical errors he made along the way and his passion to create culture that admits our fallibility as people and to establish important safeguards to protect patients from harm.

Tiny Medicine is a current book. It chronicles the progress made since the old days of practicing medicine, in which, "We actively cultivated an aura of error-free perfection and hid our mistakes from the rest of the world." Instead, through his incredibly personal and gripping narrative, Chris actively shares what it is to be human—

full of hopes, fears, and imperfections. Throughout, he opens himself, and the practice of medicine, up to us.

In this beautifully written firsthand account, we receive an unflinching glimpse behind the curtain of the day-to-day world of practicing neonatology. We discover that there are 15 million premature infants born each year. Wow. We learn how to visualize how small preemie babies actually can be—that they can weigh up to 12 times less than a full-term baby. We develop appreciation for the men and women who dedicate themselves to saving these babies' lives.

Tiny Medicine is an honest book. It is full of truths that NICU care teams face every day, but that the rest of us can only imagine, including daily run-ins with the "alphas and omegas" of life in the form of both births and deaths, sometimes hours apart. Chris shares both the awesome responsibility and actual nausea he felt on his first day as a NICU attending physician at Mission Hospital. He shares accounts of unwavering perseverance—including the story of Alyssa, who was the smallest preemie he ever treated, weighing in at 360 grams (about 3/4 of a pound) at birth, and is now a happy, rambunctious preschooler. He shares with us his many days of practice giving bad news to patients and the moment that the practice all made sense and he felt true empathy. He shares with us his somber experience filling out his first death certificate, skills that were never taught in medical school.

Tiny Medicine is an important book and should be required reading for anyone in the healthcare field. In his chapter covering quality, Chris details his own mistakes as a clinician and discusses the inevitability that doctors, as humans, will make errors. Instead of covering up these mistakes, he advocates for disclosure, root cause

Introduction

"In nothing do men more nearly approach the gods than in giving health to others."

–Cicero: *Pro Ligario XII*, 46 BC

Patients all over the world will experience an event today that divides their lives in half. Before and after the birth of a child. Before and after the death of a parent. Before and after the heart attack. Before and after cancer.

For most of us, these events are exceptionally rare. But physicians play a role in shaping them for their patients many times a day, day after day, for decades.

Medical school and residency equip us with the knowledge we need to identify and treat even the most seemingly insurmountable diagnoses, and superior clinical performance is crucial to being a great physician. What medical school doesn't do is prepare us for how a life spent repeatedly bearing witness to these inflection points in other people's lives will forever shape our own.

Imagine standing in a cramped hospital room where a premature infant is dying. He's barely 12 hours old and you've spent every one of those 12 hours trying to save his life. You have come to know his mother and father by first name and they know you by yours. Even in this short time they have grown to trust you, to depend on you, to celebrate with you, and to cry with you, all the while riding a rollercoaster of emotion. Such a turbulent trip may be unprecedented in their lives, but not in yours.

You've prepared them for this moment since the beginning, and when an hour ago the baby's blood pressure kept dropping no matter how many drugs you pumped into his pint-sized body, you told them his battle was nearly over. No matter what you or God or anyone else did next, he wasn't going to win.

You managed to keep him alive long enough for his parents to fill the room with family members crowded around in uncomfortable chairs. Grandparents, uncles, aunts, and friends all physically present but without any clue what to say or how to feel except sad.

After everyone has had a chance to hold him, nuzzle him, hug him, and kiss him, his mother brings him close to her chest. You lock eyes and share a moment that makes it clear now is the time. The rhythmic bounce of his chest stops as you gently remove his breathing tube, allowing his mother to see his face unencumbered for the first time. You both cry.

Within minutes he's lost his pulse and you place the bell of your impossibly small stethoscope on his impossibly small chest for a full sixty seconds just like you learned in medical school. With no breathing and no heartbeat, you again look up into his mother's eyes and let her know that he's gone. Time of death 2:37 a.m.

You all grieve together and then you leave the room so his family can grieve alone. In any normal universe, you'd then wake your kids up to make sure they all still have a pulse and know how much you love them and process your own sense of loss, of failure, of grief.

But you can't.

Instead your pager goes off and, without missing a beat, you run to another room where a new family is delivering another premature baby. A tiny baby girl joining the world four months before her due date and whose entire life relies on all the skill, training, and expertise you and your enormous team of partners can muster. You cannot stop—this baby and her family deserve your very best, and no matter what happened in the room you've just left, you cannot allow your best to be any less for this baby. If anything, you feel a burning need to somehow make it be more.

Physicians fool ourselves into thinking we can live like this at work, go home, and then live our lives like normal people. We think we can engage meaningfully with each individual patient while having a deep enough well to move from patient to patient, inflection point to inflection point, without carrying the weight of the last one. Or the one before that. Or the hundreds upon hundreds before that any physician faces over a 30-plus-year career. This is what the profession demands, but it comes with both incredible cost and incredible reward and fundamentally shapes and reshapes who we are as people.

We don't talk about this with our patients. We barely talk about it with each other. So I will.

Tiny Medicine is filled with stories about the ups and downs, the absurd and the sublime of caring for the world's smallest patients. The stories are centered around how becoming and being a neonatologist has continually shaped and reshaped who I am as a doctor, a husband, a father, and a person. I'll share the path I took to becoming a doctor, the secrets of life inside the neonatal intensive care unit (NICU), the loneliness that comes with a doctor's responsibility for inflection point decisions, and the powerful sense of purpose and triumph that can come from just making it through the night. You'll read stories of hope, of life and death, of good triumphing over evil, and of what it's like to plumb the bottom of a doctor's professional well.

In the end, writing this book is as much a personal journey for me as it is an effort to provide you a window into a world you may never otherwise experience: what it's really like to be a doctor fortunate enough to care for the smallest, sickest, most helpless yet often most seemingly invincible patients in the world.

One last note before sending you on. One of my patients—who is now of age to do so—and the mother of a second patient (who is decidedly still well underage) have provided their express written permission to use their real names and real stories. Their names are Stephen Kirchner, who you will meet in Chapter 6, and Alyssa Summey, who you will meet in Chapter 7. Alyssa was still a preschooler at the time of this writing, but her mother Haley provided permission. I am humbled to have played a role in their lives both inside the hospital and out, and am now doubly so in being able to share the parts of their stories that intersect with mine. All other patient names are entirely fictional and bear no intentional connection to any actual patient. Any unintentional connections are entirely coincidental, and are designated as such with an asterisk (*) next to the first time they are mentioned.

Finally, I have intentionally changed some of the times, places, ages, genders, and other small details of certain stories to completely ensure that the patients, families, and sometimes colleagues involved remain anonymous. Aside from these minor intentional changes, I also admit that time has likely rolled the stones of some of these stories around the corners of my mind enough that their edges have become smoothed. It's therefore possible that I've combined the details of one story with those of another into a composite I believe to be true but may actually be two separate episodes. For this I'll ask both your forgiveness and your indulgence.

Dr. Chris DeRienzo
Asheville, North Carolina. December 31, 2018

– 1 –

Getting There

"Mr. Spock: Doctor, if I were able to show emotion, your new infatuation with that term would begin to annoy me.

Dr. McCoy: What term? "Logic?" Medical men are trained in logic, Mr. Spock.

Mr. Spock: Really, Doctor? I had no idea they were trained. Watching you, I assumed it was trial and error."

–Leonard Nimoy and DeForest Kelley: *Star Trek*

The nausea was so overwhelming it nearly sent me to the ground. I'd spent 31 years in training if you count preschool preparing for this day, my first day as an attending physician running my own neonatal intensive care unit (NICU) service.

By that point, I'd been a doctor for six years and had made thousands of in-the-moment decisions that were only later validated by my supervising attending physician. The time had come, however, for me to take to the trapeze without a net. I no longer had a supervisor looking over my shoulder—I was the attending, and the final call on each decision was entirely my own. Just like a trapeze artist swinging without a net for the first time, the magnitude of that responsibility hit me hard, and sent my stomach reeling. After all, that responsibility was why I went into medicine in the first place, and its full weight now finally rested on my shoulders.

Truth be told, the arc of my life had bent toward medicine since I was in Underoos. When I was 5, my family lived in a small Long Island town about an hour outside of New York City. My father had torn the place down to the studs and rebuilt it into a bustling home, replete with backyard swing-set, batting tee, Slip-N-Slide, and a variety of enormous-looking bushes. I remember playing outside near those bushes with my sister one day in the middle of summer. It was her second birthday party, and the bushes were covered from top to bottom with small red berries. The kind that look just like candy to 2-year-olds.

As a firstborn genetically incapable of not serving as guardian and protector of all within my keep, I watched her walk toward the back stoop then suddenly lurch for the berries and shove a handful in her mouth. They must have been bitter, because I remember her making a terrible face, spitting them out, and then toddling off toward the Slip-N-Slide.

I took off into the house, heart pounding and hands spinning over my head like the lights on an old police car while screaming "EMERGENCY! EMERGENCY!" I relayed the story, crushed that I failed to stop her from eating the berries and convinced I would lose my first patient to backyard berry poisoning before I'd even been to kindergarten. A quick (and reassuring) call to poison control and all was returned to normal. Except for the helpless bushes, as my father slipped silently away from the party and promptly turned them into wood chips.

My mother practiced nursing before my siblings and I were born, and I grew up marveling at how much she knew about healing. She always had an answer, a treatment, a reassurance for whatever was ailing anyone in the family, and I wanted to know just as much about caring for people as she did. By the time I hit elementary school, other kids were coming to me routinely for medical advice about bug bites and scrapes. I remember one day on the playground in first grade, a boy bloodied his knee playing kickball and a flotilla of children came running my way. He had a small cut just under his kneecap that was indeed bleeding but would clearly stop on its own. I vividly remember thinking to myself, "Well, touching blood with my bare hands is risky, but I really need to treat my patient." I wiped away his blood, told everyone he'd be fine, and the group went back to playing.

Recess ended and I walked to the school nurse's office, ready to face whatever horrors awaited me for touching blood without wearing the appropriate personal protective equipment. Pale and trembling, I told the nurse what happened, and said that I was ready now for the gigantic needle I was convinced she needed to use to test me for all manner and variety of infectious diseases. She instead gave me a popsicle, reminded me that I didn't have a license to practice either nursing or medicine in the state of New York, and sent me back to class.

While I didn't know it yet, even at 8 years old, the strains of the American Medical Association's 1847 *Code of Ethics* rang true in my heart, which says a physician must be "ever ready to obey the calls of the sick... because there is no tribunal other than his own conscience, to adjudge penalties for carelessness or neglect."

While I spent years in my childhood dreaming about medicine, it turns out that the actual practice of medicine is rather different from what most people think. Centuries of folklore have given us a gilded picture of the good doctor, sitting in a dark, wood-paneled library surrounded by stack upon stack of medical textbooks. The air is heavy, and you can practically feel the weight of ancient wisdom as the ghosts of Osler, Galen, Hippocrates, and other famous physicians from history hover over his shoulders. His white coat is rumpled, reading glasses askew, and you can just make out his furrowed brow beneath the amber light of his table lamp as he desperately tries to connect the dots.

We watch for a moment as he moves from book to book, the gears in his mind spinning faster and faster until something finally catches his eye. It's a line from the 19th century Latin translation of the Ancient Egyptian *Ebers Papyrus* and it sends him headlong again into the stacks. Thousand-page tomes by Sabiston and Harrison crash thunderously to the floor until he finally emerges with a copy of *Nelson's Textbook of Pediatrics*. Rifling through the pages, he stops on page 1,754, scans the minuscule print, pounds his fist against the heavy wooden desk so hard it startles the medical students hunched in their nearby cubbies, and exclaims, "Of course!"

He grabs the book and streaks down the Gothic library corridors, his white coat a blur as he bursts through the hospital's main doors and re-enters its cold, sterile embrace. Taking the stairs two at a time, he climbs five flights up to the pediatric ward. Stopping only briefly at the pharmacy, he sprints to his patient's room, locks eyes with the young girl's parents, and with both relief and triumph in his face says, "We've got it."

He starts an intravenous line in her tiny arm, spikes the clear glass bottle of medication, opens the clamp and the mysterious drug begins flowing into her bloodstream. Within a matter of seconds, her eyelids flutter, she begins to stir, the corners of her mouth curl into a weak smile and she opens her eyes for the first time in days. Her parents rejoice while the good doctor slumps into an uncomfortable rocking chair, the weight of one life lifted from his shoulders.

Medicine is practiced like this in exactly two places: 19th century British paintings and prime-time television dramas.

My real life as a physician has never been so simple. While like any doctor I've had a handful of "eureka" moments, I can't count the number of times I've fallen asleep on hard call-room mattresses thinking about a particularly challenging patient and woken up still thinking, struggling to find the one unifying diagnosis that would perfectly connect all the dots.

Real medicine is messier than it looks in paintings or on television, diagnoses are rarely perfectly cut and dried, and with the possible exception of doctors old enough to have actually used glass bottles and metal IV catheters, you should almost never allow a doctor to start your IV. We're just not as good at it as nurses are, a fact my wife (an oncology nurse) finds reason to remind me of nearly every day.

My first chance to experience the complex choreography of real medicine came as a teenager living in a bucolic Massachusetts town about 45 minutes west of Boston. I was incredibly fortunate to have Dr. Mary-Ellen Taplin as a neighbor, a world-class cancer doctor who introduced me to the wonders of science and medicine through her oncology research. She took me into her lab one summer and showed me what cancer looks like under the microscope. She explained how she was trying to isolate specific genes responsible for changing normal prostate cells into the rapidly dividing monsters that grow into tumors. While all of the then state-of-the-art pipetting, polymerase chain reaction, and DNA blotting experiments we ran in her lab were fascinating, what I found most exciting were our trips to the tumor board.

Tumor boards are clinical meetings where all of the cancer-treating experts in the hospital—surgeons, oncologists, radiologists, pathologists, research scientists, and more—collect to weigh in on the most challenging cancer patients' cases. These weren't teaching cases or research cases—these were real patients, real people with real doctors all working together to make really hard decisions about how best to treat them. The complexity was titanic. The teamwork was inspiring. The mantle was daunting. I decided then and there in our last tumor board of the summer that I would go to medical school.

I went to college just outside of Boston, and during my freshman year I wanted to get as close as I could to really treating patients. I took an emergency medical technician (EMT) course offered by the campus EMT squad and passed the exam in the spring of 2000. I spent the next three years volunteering as a campus EMT, responding to calls for everything from seizures to car wrecks to drunks. Lots, and lots, and lots of drunks.

In my junior year, I remember getting a 911 call for a kid who was convinced his tongue was alive. He was flailing around in the middle of the lawn between two large dormitories, terrified that his tongue was literally going to crawl out of his mouth. I channeled both my mother and the school nurse from first grade while trying my best to reassure him that, no matter how much tequila one drinks, tongues cannot independently detach from a human's mouth.

I had a fantastic time working as an EMT, both for the university squad and for a local 911 and non-emergency ambulance service. I also supplemented my time on ambulances with a job in our local hospital's emergency department as a technician during summers back home. Really connecting with patients one-on-one for the first time fueled me through the countless hours of organic chemistry, physics, and biochemistry required to pass the medical school entrance exam. It also gave me an abundance of stories to tell medical school admissions deans, who read thousands of such stories every year in the application essays of aspiring medical students. My essay about performing CPR wound up being intriguing enough to land interviews around the country. Having fallen head over heels for North Carolina's warm spring and ready to finally escape New England winters, in June of 2003 I found myself driving 12 hours south to Durham, North Carolina to begin my career as a doctor at the Duke University School of Medicine.

Medical School

From the very first day in medical school, medical students are taught that there are only two diagnoses we'll never make in our careers: the diagnosis we don't know about and the diagnosis we don't think about. This experience is made manifest in a medical student's introductory visit to the medical school bookstore getting ready for Day 1 of the "basic science" lectures.

I'd bought a lot of textbooks in college, but that first day in the Medical School Bookstore convinced me that the authors of medical textbooks must be paid by the word. I brought home at least five multi-volume sets, each with pages numbering well into the thousands. I was in fairly good shape at the time for a 22-year-old, but I needed reinforced cardboard boxes and a thick-wheeled hand-truck to get the bloated corpus into my apartment.

Once you really get down to it, the most daunting part of medical school isn't the ingestion of tens of thousands of pages of medical knowledge. In those first few months, we had hundreds of pages of reading each week across different textbooks interspersed with hour after hour of PowerPoint lectures and microscope time looking at pre-prepared slides. We also had the occasional exam that required you to regurgitate back reams of information in order to prove that you had really ingested it. This is where medical school differs most from college.

In college, finals week for me involved many, many hours of memorization, followed by one final and a massive explosion of knowledge aimed into the pages of a wide-ruled exam book, followed inevitably by the immediate liberation from my brain of everything I'd just memorized to make room for the next exam's batch. The cycle repeated itself, binging and purging course after course of knowledge, one exam so different from the next that there was rarely a need to remember the content after passing the final exam.

Medicine doesn't work that way. In order to practice medicine, you need to deeply understand pathophysiology, which is the science of all the ways in which the functions of the human body can go terribly wrong. Once you truly understand pathophysiology, you can then systematically work through all the ways you can try to fix the things that can go wrong, pick the best, and treat your patient. However, in order to understand pathophysiology, you have to understand physiology, microbiology, immunology, and pharmacology, and in order to understand those, you have to know anatomy, biochemistry, molecular biology, and cell biology. Each step builds upon the last, and like a teetering Jenga tower, you can't skimp on the base without endangering the penthouse. Figuring this out was, by far, the most overwhelming part of my first year in medical school— knowing that if I ever fell behind there would be no chance to catch back up.

In order to survive the year, I had to completely break down and build back up my approach to learning, which I suppose is in fact the point. Doctors must be lifelong learners, and medical school prepares our brains to continually add new Jenga blocks over the course of our careers while replacing old ones to keep pace with the exponentially expanding universe of medical information. This gets easier when each new bit of knowledge is connected to a real person, a story in which you have personally played a role. That's what practicing clinical medicine is like, but you don't get there until you've run the first-year basic science gauntlet.

If the basic science courses in medical school re-taught me how to learn, the rest of medical school re-taught me how to think. Learning the language of clinical medicine restructures the way your brain thinks about the world and fundamentally shapes how a doctor approaches treating patients. In the clinical years of medical school, I was taught how to take a history, how to perform a physical exam, and how to integrate the signs and symptoms of one with the other to construct a logically consistent story of a patient's state of health.

Once we learn how to extract every bit of information we can from a patient through conversation, observation, and examination, medical school teaches doctors to progress through a phase called "the differential diagnosis." As medical students, we were expected to actually write out this thought experiment, the post-graduate equivalent of a fourth-grade math student asked to show her work when performing double-digit multiplication. Having weighed all the possible causes for a patient's constellation of signs, symptoms, laboratory findings, and radiology findings, it is then time to put down your chips and make a call. You write a statement known as your "assessment"—e.g., this is a 2-year-old boy with fever, right ear pain, and pus behind his ear drum, who most likely has an acute bacterial otitis media (an ear infection). Finally, you commit to your "plan," which in this case would include some combination of antibiotics, acetaminophen, ibuprofen, and advice that his parents sleep while they can because they're in for a few days of total misery.

We practiced writing these observations over and over again in student "History and Physical" notes, documents that never became part of the medical record and instead were submitted to our attending physicians for review. They read them with gusto and an active red pen, grading us as much on our thinking as on our writing and watching with pride as the expansive and disconnected H&P of a second-year medical student slowly but surely transitions into the tight, well-reasoned narrative of a fourth-year.

During these clinical years of medical school, budding doctors are also introduced to the panoply of medical and surgical subspecialties. Everyone rotates through core clerkships in surgery, internal medicine, pediatrics, psychiatry, family medicine, and obstetrics and gynecology (OB-GYN). In just those few weeks, medical students sample what the next 40 years might feel like—and the arc of a doctor's life looks very, very different specialty by specialty.

I started my clinical year on surgery, widely acknowledged among my peers as the hardest clerkship and the best to "get out of the way" early on. Pre-rounds with the residents—a ritual in all hospitals where trainees visit the wards to check on their patients before actual rounds with the supervising attending later in the day—started at 6 a.m. This meant that medical students who wanted to know something about their patients to present to the interns in pre-rounds had to be at work well before then to pre-pre-round.

When I started medical school, the world of hospital and clinic medicine was all still paper-based, so I would hit the wards before 5 a.m. and begin gathering information like vital sign trends and overnight changes from my patients' paper charts, logging it all on a printed patient list. I'd then talk to the nightshift nurses to get the insider-intel, gleaning portions of the patient's story that would never make it into their notes. Finally, I'd quietly see the patients myself and examine their surgical wounds. By 5:30 I'd be back in the medical student lounge rehearsing how to present the information to the residents at 6 a.m.

At 6 a.m., the team assembled, consisting of two to three medical students and at least four residents. One, the intern in his first year of surgical training after completing medical school, was responsible for running the service and manning the service pager. I spent two weeks with him and that pager never went more than seven minutes without beeping day and night, weekday and weekend. The second resident, called a JAR (short for Junior Assistant Resident), actually got to see the inside of the operating room from time to time and served as the intern's immediate backup. The SAR, or Senior Assistant Resident, was backup for the JAR and spent most of her time in the operating room beginning to perfect the procedural nature of her craft. Then there was the Chief, a resident in his final year of surgical training, who ran the team and was the direct conduit to the attending surgeons whose patients we covered across the hospital's wards.

My Chief on that first two-week clerkship was one of the best I would rotate with through all of medical school. He knew the particular idiosyncrasies of each attending surgeon, some of whom enjoying drilling medical students on the histories of particular surgical procedures and others who preferred their medical students silent at all times. When we'd present on pre-rounds, he used to tell medical students to "Speak like I'm holding a match in my hand. If you aren't done before the match burns my finger, you're toast." He was only half kidding.

A typical pre-rounds presentation, back at the patient's bedside but this time with an army of short white coats filling the room and protruding out the door and into the hallway, sounded something like this:

"Mr. J is now post-operative day 2 from his right hemi-colectomy. His vitals were stable overnight, he is now passing flatus and tolerated his liquid diet. His abdomen is non-tender, his surgical site is clean, dry, and intact, and he feels well this morning. I would like to advance his diet, get him out of bed as tolerated, and transition him to oral medications." Physicians love their jargon, and this jargon-filled paragraph more or less translates to: "He had surgery to take out half of his intestines two days ago, but whatever intestines are left are moving again because he's farting and his belly doesn't hurt, so it's time to get him ready to go home."

If you got it right, the Chief would nod in general agreement, exchanging pleasantries with the patient while performing a brief physical exam himself, and then rapidly move on.

When I wasn't the medical student responsible for presenting a particular patient, my job was to man the chart. I'd run ahead of the white coat phalanx to the next patient's room, pull down the door cabinet, flip open the chart and find the next blank space for the intern to begin writing orders. Once pre-rounds for the patient were complete, I'd have to close the chart, toss it into the rolling chair we carried behind us on rounds, and run to the next room in advance of the armada so as not to grind the entire process to a halt. After finishing pre-rounds on the unit, we would stop by the front desk, drop off all the charts with new orders written inside them into an enormous chart bucket, and then run back ahead of the team to get to the next unit

Since running is frowned upon in hospital hallways unless there's a real emergency, I learned how to walk very fast. I'm not a tall person, but if you stride far enough and with a quick-enough cadence I learned that I could outwalk an intern who looks like he should be playing center for the Boston Celtics. To this day people ask me why I walk so fast, and I tell them I'm still recovering from my medical school surgery clerkship, forever in my mind hearing the howling of a thousand

Dansko medical clogs pounding the laminate floors of Duke Hospital behind me.

There were parts of surgery I really enjoyed, including how seemingly definitively we could fix problems like fractured bones, infected appendices, and hernias. Patients were genuinely grateful that they came in with something broken and left with whatever it was more or less fixed. And the operating room is something of a sacred space, where even amidst the rock music and team banter there are inviolable rules akin to church practices that evoke an aura of the rare and divine.

That said, the prospect of an alarm clock set at 3:45 a.m. for the rest of my life and having to spend nearly another decade in training before getting to ply my craft were not appealing. Nor were some aspects of surgery itself—I once spent nearly an hour leaning backwards from the operating room table holding an illuminated anal retractor for a particularly grumpy rectal surgeon. He kept repositioning my hands, saying "you aren't holding the light right" until finally grabbing the thing himself and swearing about how medical students "never knew what the f--- they were doing." I wanted to scream back, "No kidding man, that's why it's called medical SCHOOL" but bit my tongue. Lying in bed that night, I reckoned that if I spent 12 hours a day for 30 years staring through magnifying lenses into other people's butts, I would probably be perpetually grumpy too.

My surgery clerkship was also the first and so far only time that I've stuck myself with a needle. It happened near the end of my two-week block with the orthopedic surgeons as we were finishing a total hip replacement on a very elderly gentleman. The major part of the procedure was done, which involved sawing off the end of the man's thigh bone (also called the femur), replacing it with a metal implant, and hammering the shiny new hip into the carcass of the old one. We were now just closing the wound with sutures, a medical student's job and one I'd done several times before.

I was using a suture needle so big it looked like a fish hook to close the outermost muscle covering, doing my best to get the tissues as close together as possible to promote rapid healing. Three quarters of the way through, I was using my fingers to bring together the farthest edges of the wound when I turned the suture needle a hair too far and passed it right through my double-gloves and into my index finger. I immediately removed the instruments from the sterile field, announced to the resident I'd stuck myself and stepped back from the table, face pale as a ghost. I broke scrub and went to the sink, praying I'd only felt the poke through the first layer of gloves and wouldn't be bleeding underneath. I was.

I left the operating room and dragged myself to employee health, where they drew my labs to determine if I needed to take any chemoprophylaxis against HIV or Hepatitis C. The needle they used to take my blood wasn't nearly as huge as the one my first-grade self had imagined, but the level of anxiety was the same.

The hospital did not require consent to test a patient's blood for the presence of HIV or Hepatitis when a clinician was stuck, so they sent some of his "extra" blood already in the lab for testing and said they would call me when it was back. While an octogenarian receiving a hip replacement was about as low risk a patient to get stuck by as it gets, the 12 hours I spent waiting for that call were agonizingly long. When I got the call, they said both his labs and mine were normal, and while it was remotely possible that he was in a "window" phase where he'd contracted one of these viruses but wasn't yet showing symptoms of them, the odds were vanishingly small. I was free to return to suturing at will, and while I've sewn countless central lines into newborns' umbilical cords, I've never again tried to sew up a hip.

In addition to catching the transition from paper to electronic medical records, my time in medical school predated "work hour restrictions" for medical students but directly coincided with their introduction for residents. This meant that while residents were at least on paper limited to working no more than 80 hours a week averaged over a full month and required to have at least one day off each week, medical students were not. As a result, with residency programs trying to figure out how to run hospital services with the same number of residents available for fewer hours, medical students were sometimes leaned on to pick up the slack.

The work of a medical student on any rotation was more or less the same and within medicine is referred to as "scut" work. Scut work is a catch-all term for all of the administrative tasks required to run a hospital service that no one wants to deal with. Thus, they keep falling down the food chain and land with a thud on the medical student's head. Even senior medical students, rotating as "acting interns" on hospital services would "scut out" their more junior second-year colleagues, asking them to run tubes of blood to the lab, call a nursing home to get a patient's long and detailed medical history, label a full stack of blank progress notes with each patient's sticker to facilitate the following day's work, and so on. Ostensibly this kind of work was somehow connected to "learning," but beyond discovering the most efficient way to sort and sticker paper, I'm not sure how it made me a better doctor.

While always the purview of trainees, this kind of scut work shifted heavily into medical students' laps after the onset of resident work hour restrictions. There was simply no longer enough time in a resident's day to finish everything she was expected to do. On surgery, this meant getting in early and staying late each day with the saving grace of one full day off each week. I spent those off days largely sleeping, recovering from the 90 hours I'd just worked, and re-energizing for the next onslaught of 18-hour challenges.

As the bright colors of fall gave way to the grays of winter, I finished my surgery clerkship and moved on to internal medicine. At least the grueling hours of surgery held the promise of one recovery day each week—such was not the case on medicine. At the time, medical students on their medicine rotations were allotted two days off a month, expected to come into the hospital "as early as required," and expected to stay "as late as required" as many nights as required to get our jobs done. As luck would have it, I used up my only two days off that first month for an American Medical Association leadership meeting, which meant spending some portion of 26 days straight in the hospital.

Internists have a fundamentally different approach to practicing medicine than surgeons. Instead of whipping through rounds from bedside to bedside with matchstick speed to get to the operating room for a 7:30 a.m. first case start, rounds on internal medicine lasted for hours. In the years before patient-centered bedside rounding, internal medicine rounds involved sitting around a conference room table talking through every possible diagnosis a patient could be suffering from before finally settling on a plan for the day. As medical students, we had a solemn duty to keep each other from falling asleep, failing only in the rare circumstance that the foreheads of both medical students assigned to the service hit the table simultaneously.

Often the discussion veered far away from the actual patient and deep into the theoretical, with the attending physician asking questions like "Medical Student Chris, if this patient had presented with itchy skin and a mild yellowing in his eyes instead of right-sided abdominal pain that worsened whenever he breathed in, what would you move to the top of your differential diagnosis list?" These discussions were far different from Dr. Taplin's tumor boards I'd so cherished in high school—instead of solving problems, they pitted students and residents against the attending's seemingly endless font of medical knowledge until it was clear he would forget more about some esoteric subject (like thyroid pathophysiology) than we could ever hope to learn. I'm sure these rounds worked well for some, but for me they were torture.

I spent the last two weeks of that 26-day stretch caring for a full service of patients who had all made poor health decisions and were either actively dying or passively dying and didn't realize it yet. My patients included smokers with lung cancer permeating nearly every corner of their bodies, alcoholics with liver failure so bad they wouldn't survive long enough to qualify for a transplant, and IV drug users whose HIV had long ago bloomed into full-blown AIDS and whose bodies were so emaciated their skin hung like drapes on a broken window frame.

It took every ounce of emotional energy I had to care for people whose one-time preventable deaths would be wrought by their own unhealthy choices. Some patients are just incredibly unlucky; they fall and fracture their hip, get hit by a bus while crossing the street, or are randomly struck with inoperable brain cancer. Not these folks—these people had (at least at one time) intentionally made decisions, bad decisions that came back to roost in the form of devastatingly debilitating chronic—and ultimately fatal—disease. They didn't have to die like this, but now they were going to anyway.

I had entered medical school wanting to practice interventional cardiology, bringing patients to the cardiac catheterization lab to reopen their arteries and save them from death during a massive heart attack. After working 12 hours a day for 26 days straight on internal medicine, and recognizing I'd have to survive the same fate for three full years of residency before being able to train in adult cardiology, I decided I needed to find another option. I knew that to be the kind of doctor I wanted to be, I had to find a specialty that would by its very nature consistently refill my well of compassion, and that would not be adult internal medicine.

Later that spring, I met my wife while I was on my OB-GYN rotation. I had the best Chief Resident in the history of the hospital leading my gynecology oncology service, the only other service in a medical student's career that required a 3:45 a.m. wake-up call. We had been on service together for about a week, and around noon on a Tuesday he looked me in the eye and said, "Christopher, you are a fantastic medical student, you work hard and deserve some down time. Give me your pager and go take a two-hour lunch break." My eyes shot open and before he could change his mind, I thanked him profusely, handed him my pager, and sped off the ward toward 120 minutes of mid-day freedom.

Medical students have a preternatural ability to sense

free food anywhere in the hospital, and that day I was no exception. I followed my nose down to the lecture halls on the hospital's second floor, where there was a talk in the main hall accompanied by a free lunch open to medical students. An author was speaking, and it just so happened that it was the same author whose mandatory lecture I'd skipped in college. I thought to myself this was karma smacking me upside the head, and started to head toward the lunch line. That's when I saw what the other lecture hall had planned for the day.

Outside of the smaller room to the right of the main hall was a table filled with a second platter of free food and copies of a book written by a double-amputee who had climbed Mount Kilimanjaro. Surrounding that table and spilling out into the foyer was a crowd of nursing students. My eyes met those of one particularly attractive nursing student standing near the front of the table and wearing a white patterned scrub top and navy pants. She was standing with a few other nursing students and smiled when she saw me. The first thought that hit my brain was "Whoa." The second was "What the hell, Chris, give it a shot." I walked up to her and introduced myself, and we chatted while she worked her way through her lunch line. Not wanting to stop our conversation, I asked her to save me a seat in her lecture hall and said I would sneak out of mine as soon as I could to join her and her friends. She agreed.

I got my lunch and found one of my best friends sitting in the back row of the medical students' hall. I said, "Eric, there's a nursing student saving me a seat next door—cover for me if someone notices I left." He said I was full of cow excrement but he'd do his best. As soon as the author took the stage, I snuck over the back row of chairs, shuffled past a cluster of sleeping medical students, and silently exited the room. Sure enough, there in the very back row in the very back corner was my nursing student, saving me a seat. I have absolutely no memory of what the amputee discussed, my attention instead fixed to a pair of blue-green eyes unlike any I'd ever seen before. We've been together ever since.

That summer I hit my block on the pediatrics service and finally found my home as a physician. The hours were still long, yet everyone on every team from doctors and nurses to technicians and unit clerks acted just a little bit different than those on the adult services. The Duke Children's Hospital took up almost the entire fifth floor of Duke's main bed tower. Across that floor we took care of all kinds of children. Some were born with heart disease and survived multiple run-ins with the operating room as surgeons reconstructed their hearts and major associated blood vessels. Now they ran around the unit playing freeze tag, their heart disease palliated just enough to last into adulthood and secure an easier chance of finding a donor for a heart transplant. We had children born without immune systems hidden behind double-locked doors and accessible only through a guarded ante room. Still others were in various stages of battling cancer, all just a few rooms down from otherwise healthy children admitted with pneumonia, asthma attacks, and skin infections.

My pediatric rotation also included time in the outpatient clinics, where I saw everything from happy and healthy kids for their annual well-checks to the pediatric equivalent of every subspecialty in adult medicine—pediatric cardiology, pediatric endocrinology, pediatric oncology, and more. What struck me more than anything else, though, was how easy it was for me to maintain my well of compassion while treating kids. Absolutely nothing that happened to these patients (save perhaps a few older kids on the adolescent service) was their fault, and for some reason that kept my emotional resiliency balanced enough to weather the inevitable downsides of caring for children. Every doctor is different and I have nothing but respect for surgeons, internists, psychiatrists, and OB-GYNs, but after six weeks on my pediatric clerkship I knew without a doubt that I was going to be a pediatrician.

The rest of medical school was a blur of elective rotations and "acting internships." During Duke's mandatory research year, I attended the Terry Sanford School of Public Policy and secured a master's degree. I also spent two years on the American Medical Association's Board of Trustees, got married, and interviewed all over the country for a residency position in pediatrics. On the day of the residency match—where a magical algorithm running on a server farm somewhere outside of Washington matches medical students' rank-order program lists with each program's rank-order student lists—I opened my envelope and was fortunate to stay at Duke.

When you don't have to uproot your life and move across the country, the last six weeks of medical school are a magical time. Friends of mine who had unexpectedly matched in far-away programs were desperately trying to rent or sell their homes, find a mover, and find a new place to live near whatever hospital they'd be more or less living in as residents. By matching and staying at Duke I had none of those problems—instead, I had six weeks of simply not getting expelled from school standing between me and finally being a doctor.

Graduation day came on May 9, 2008. That night in a dark, wood-paneled room just after 8 p.m., I joined

89 other medical students all freshly adorned with the ceremonial green academic hoods of medicine in reciting the Hippocratic Oath. In pictures from that evening you can see a combination of intense pride and profound nausea in my wife's eyes as she battled morning sickness in the eighth week of pregnancy with our oldest daughter. In my parent's eyes, there's relief that their son had chosen a relatively stable career path combined with the additional relief that I'd be unlikely to move back home any time soon. My eyes tell a different story from picture to picture. In some, there's a combination of purpose and joy that only those who've found their calling in life can truly express. In others, the halting reprieve of a ship's captain having successfully navigated through the crest of one massive wave while the heft of the next slowly builds before his eyes.

No matter. I was finally a doctor.

– 2 –

Tiny Medicine

"Don't give up! I believe in you all.
A person's a person, no matter how small!"

–Horton (Dr. Seuss): *Horton Hears a Who*

When I tell people I'm a neonatologist, they usually nod and smile in the awkward way people do when they have absolutely no idea what you're talking about. I've learned to follow this up with "you know, the kind of a doctor who takes care of really small and really sick NICU babies." Most people's eyes then immediately brighten as they identify with a niece, cousin, or friend whose baby had to stay in the NICU for a couple of days. Then they invariably talk about how amazing the nurses were and how small the other NICU babies were in nearby isolettes.

Premature infants are small. Very small. They're so small that our normal physical understanding of the world just doesn't make sense. Calling them "small" is like describing a galaxy as "big" or the sun as "heavy." Words simply cannot do the real thing justice.

If you really want to grasp NICU small—and you're

not up for volunteering in your local NICU as a cuddler—you're going to need some props. I recommend that you put down this book, go to your kitchen, and get a gallon of milk, a soda can, a straw, a spoon, and a grape.

Start by picking up the milk. A full gallon of milk weighs plus or minus 8½ pounds, varying just a flicker whether you prefer slightly heavier whole milk or the slightly lighter skim variety. Close your eyes and really feel the weight, imagining a newborn crying in your arms while you gently rock her back and forth. An average newborn actually weighs just a little less than the gallon of milk (closer to 7 pounds), but two of my three kids weighed more than the gallon you're holding, so it's a close enough approximation for our purposes.

Now transfer the gallon of milk to one hand and pick up the soda can with the other. In America, most soda cans contain 12 ounces of your favorite carbonated sugary beverage, which (including the mass of the aluminum can itself) weighs about the same as the smallest NICU babies I've cared for as a doctor. An adult's weight fluctuates more than 12 ounces—or just under 400 grams—over the course of just a few hours. Yet 400 grams is more than enough to contain the sum total of the smallest person I've ever met. You'll get to meet her in Chapter 7.

Imagine the contrast as you walk down a hallway in the NICU, passing the soda-can-sized baby hunkered down in her isolette (also called an incubator), sandwiched between two giant infants of diabetic mothers, each over 12 times her size. To put this massive size discrepancy in perspective, if I was next to another human being 12 times as big as me, he would stand 72 feet tall or about the length of an average blue whale. He would also weigh nearly a ton and his palm could fit me, my wife, and my three kids all lying together in a line head-to-foot while still being able to close his fingers in a fist. It shouldn't then be a surprise that caring for babies 12 times smaller than other newborns requires really, really tiny medicine.

Now put down the drinks and pick up the straw. Most grocery store drinking straws have an interior diameter of about 6 millimeters, or just a quarter of an inch. (Yes, I actually measured a sample of straws for the sole purpose of this comparison.) I want you to pick up the straw and look through its hole—hold it really close to your eye, and try to really appreciate how hard it would be to breathe through such a tiny passageway. Despite incredible advances in care over the past century, the smallest and most premature babies invariably need a breathing tube and specialized high-frequency ventilators for some period of time to support their immature lungs. The breathing tubes that doctors and other providers use in the NICU to intubate their windpipes have an interior diameter of only 2.5 millimeters. You could easily fit two of them inside the straw you're looking through with room to spare.

Learning to intubate babies this small was one of the most harrowing experiences I've had as a doctor. For obvious reasons, only the most seasoned providers are called upon to place such a tiny breathing tube in such a tiny baby, usually only seconds after the infant is born and only moments after cutting the umbilical cord. I first learned how to intubate on larger babies during residency under very controlled circumstances and with exceptionally close supervision. It wasn't until my NICU fellowship that I was given an opportunity to intubate a preemie.

Imagine holding a tube half the size of the straw in your right hand while using a glorified spoon with a flashlight on its tip to open a baby's mouth and peer inside. You're looking for a structure no bigger than the tube you're holding—the vocal cords, which look like thin white strips of dental floss standing out against the back of the baby's flesh-colored throat. To slide the tube through the cords you have to time it just right, catching the baby just as she's breathing and not trying to cry, while doing your level best not to push too hard or accidently bounce off the vocal cords and dip into the esophagus (the food pipe) that lives right below the trachea (the windpipe).

Providers are downright religious about how they prepare breathing tubes and the stylets placed inside of them to give the flexible tubes a temporarily more rigid shape. Some believe that a perfectly straight breathing tube is best, while others curve the stylet to give the breathing tube a shape reminiscent of a crescent moon. Personally, I've always been a fan of the "hockey stick" bend, which looks exactly like it sounds with a gentle curve at the top followed by a sharp bend up toward the tip that looks like you could use it to whack a microscopic puck. Since most of the tiny babies' vocal cords I've found are toward the front of their throats, using the hockey stick bend allowed me to gently rotate the tube into place along the side of a baby's mouth while maintaining the ability to still see where it's going in a space no bigger than a marble.

Should you succeed in passing the tube gently through the cords, you then have to*f* pinch the tube with your right hand, drop the laryngoscope blade from your left, very carefully pull out the stylet, and connect the tube to the respirator without moving it more than a millimeter. Should you inadvertently move it 2 millimeters, the tube might slip out of the windpipe and either drop into the esophagus or fall into the back of the baby's throat, meaning you have to start the process all over again. Oh, and you have exactly 30 seconds to complete the entire process from start to finish or risk the baby dropping her heart rate or her oxygen saturation levels. It's a high-wire act for even the most experienced intubators, especially on the tiniest of tiny babies.

Now put down the straw and pick up the spoon. Like straws, spoons vary greatly in size but a standard teaspoon can hold about 5 milliliters of liquid. Open your soda can and very carefully fill up the spoon. You may actually need to use the straw to very slowly drip it in.

When the smallest NICU babies need a blood transfusion, we give them about 10 milliliters (or 2 teaspoons) of packed red blood cells for every kilogram of their body weight. That tiny sip of soda you're holding in the teaspoon—barely enough of a taste to hazard a guess on the brand of carbonated sweetness that's in the can—is more than the amount of blood a 400-gram baby receives in each blood transfusion. And because we transfuse blood extremely slowly to protect extremely premature infants from a host of potential problems that could come from transfusing it too fast, that single teaspoon takes nearly four hours to complete its trip into the baby's bloodstream. At a speed of give or take 1 milliliter an hour, the blood is at such a high risk of clotting during the transfusion that we routinely need to place an extra intravenous line somewhere in a preemie's body to avoid losing her main intravenous lifeline for medications, hydration, and nutrition.

Presuming you're an average-sized human adult, you probably have around a thousand teaspoons of blood flowing through your heart, lungs, and bloodstream right now. A 400-gram baby has approximately 7, meaning the now minimally emptier soda can you're holding still has enough liquid to replace the baby's entire blood volume 10 times over with almost an ounce to spare. Preemies this small often need many transfusions over the course of their NICU stay, both to make up for the blood we have to draw to test their labs and to support their bone marrow, which doesn't pick up its own pace of red blood cell production for several weeks after birth. Each time you donate blood, the single unit you give (once fully processed) yields about 300 milliliters of packed red blood cells, enough to fully replace more than eight 400-gram babies' entire blood volumes or give 75 of them one transfusion.

Finally, put down the spoon and place your right hand on your heart. With your left hand, pick up the grape and carefully make a fist, closing the grape gently within your left palm. An average adult human's heart is about the size of its owner's fist and beats 70 times per minute. Look down at your left hand and imagine your own heart beating, feeling its rhythmic thump inside your chest against your right hand.

Now open your left hand. The heart of a 400-gram baby is smaller than your grape, yet contains exactly the same atria, ventricles, valves, and vessels and works in almost exactly the same way as the heart you feel now pounding against your right hand. What's more, despite its incomprehensibly small size, a preemie's heart beats on average well over 160 times per minute. This is why it takes so many adult hearts to care for just one NICU baby, and these extraordinarily small humans touch nearly every grown-up heart in the NICU during their many, many month-long stays.

Even with a good set of props, NICU small is something you truly cannot appreciate until you see it, feel it, and live it in person. I truly had absolutely no appreciation for what NICU small meant before I went to medical school. I thought I did—my younger brother was born around four weeks premature, and at under 5 pounds he seemed tiny when my parents finally brought him home from the hospital a few days after my mom was discharged. He had some yellowing of his skin, known as jaundice, and we kept his bassinet by the picture window in the front of our suburban New York home. For years I was afraid that even the slightest bump would break him into pieces.

That changed when I went to medical school. As a second-year medical student, I remember briefly setting foot in the NICU while on my pediatric surgery rotation. Everything about the place seemed intimidating. First of all, unlike other hospital units, every doctor was stopped at the front door by someone who forced you to remove your white coat, put on a hospital gown, and wash your hands up to your elbows for a full minute. Even the Chairman of the Pediatrics Department didn't get a pass—anyone who didn't spend 100% of their time in the NICU wasn't considered "clean" enough to get past the formidable head unit clerk without a thorough decontamination.

On this particular occasion, after our mandatory disinfection, my team of other medical students and surgical residents throttled through the NICU in typical surgeon fashion. We passed row upon row of isolettes, seeking the relatively large baby in whom we'd placed a gastrostomy tube—a specialized feeding tube that allows the team to pump nutrition directly into a baby's stomach—the day before. We finally found the baby, the most senior surgical resident examined his new G-tube, and upon finding everything to be healing satisfactorily we hightailed it out of there as fast as possible.

The NICU is simultaneously an intentionally intimidating place to outsiders and an incredibly welcoming place for those who enter its folds as family. I'd experienced the former—born out of an overwhelmingly parental need to protect the smallest, sickest, most vulnerable patients in the hospital—as a medical student. I'd learn the power of the latter soon enough.

My wife was pregnant with our first child when I started residency. I worked an enormous number of hours over the first six months of residency, covering different inpatient services, outpatient clinics, oncology, the general pediatrics wards, and cardiology. But thankfully I didn't reach the NICU until well after my wife gave birth in late December. I don't know how we would have made it through her first pregnancy knowing just enough about preemies to be dangerous but not enough to really understand prematurity after being exposed to how terribly things could go wrong during pregnancy without any warning. While that reality made it easy for me to practice medicine with a seemingly endless well of compassion for both mothers and babies, it would fundamentally change my appreciation for how lucky we were that everything went well for us. Fortunately, Reese was born healthy, on time, and didn't have to visit the NICU, and we had a month of an easy elective rotation to get to know our first baby.

Somewhat ironically, my first real rotation back on service the month after Reese was born was the well-baby nursery. I spent four weeks partnered with another intern and a general pediatrician seeing 25-30 healthy newborns a day, churning through reams of paperwork, and learning very little. Sometimes we'd need to bring babies who were breathing fast or having a hard time feeding into the nursery to monitor them, and a few times I had to call the NICU fellow to come take a look at a baby who wasn't turning the corner. I was incredibly intrigued with what happened once a NICU fellow decided the baby needed to go across the hallway, through the double doors and into the NICU's all-encompassing embrace. As luck would have it, my next rotation would finally bring me into the NICU on service, so I was about to find out.

I hit my first real NICU block as a doctor in the spring of my intern year. Interns—or doctors in the first year of their residency programs following medical school—have to learn quickly to imbibe from the firehose of supplemental medical knowledge needed to focus their careers on a single specialty. By then I'd been an intern for nearly nine months, and had drunk enough from the firehose to have more or less figured out everything there was to know about being a pediatrics resident anywhere else in the hospital. The NICU, however, isn't "any other rotation." As I'd briefly learned in medical school, it's a world entirely unto its own replete with a completely different vocabulary. Where else would anyone talk about "post-menstrual age" or calculate a person's weight gain in grams per day?

Along with the new vocabulary comes a new set of very specific and unyielding rules. Some of those rules, like the militant hand-washing before entering, seemed silly but were both easy to remember and easy to follow. Other rules were clinically complex, much harder to remember, and sometimes diametrically opposed to rules pounded into my brain on every other pediatric service. For example, fluid resuscitation with intravenous saline is the mainstay treatment for patients with dangerously low blood pressure anywhere else in the hospital. In the NICU, however, treating low blood pressure with aggressive intravenous fluids under anything but extraordinarily specific circumstances could create such a rapid fluid shift inside a premature infant's brain that it might burst his fragile brain's blood vessels and cause a massive brain hemorrhage. With rules like these, "Yikes" doesn't even begin to describe what an intern feels on Day 1 of a NICU block.

I will never forget the very first time I examined a real premature baby as an intern in the NICU that spring. I'd done everything required of an intern—I wore the dark blue scrubs that allowed insiders to bypass donning a hospital gown, very publicly washed my hands up to my elbows for a full minute, left my papers on the nurse's bedside stand, washed my hands again, and put on gloves. Because this baby weighed less than 1 kilogram (about 2 pounds) and was less than 2 weeks old, his skin was so fragile that no one was allowed to touch him without wearing gloves. I asked the nurse if I could examine him, and she gently helped flip him and his breathing equipment from his tummy to his back.

You may be wondering why the preemie was on his tummy when pediatricians unfailingly teach parents to put their babies "back to sleep" when they go home from the hospital. Firstly, because he was connected to a host of wires and sensors that tracked every aspect of his bodily function, which made the risk of a sudden, unwitnessed death associated with SIDS very low. Secondly, because research shows that it's actually easier for premature infants' very premature lungs to work when lying on their bellies (and appropriately monitored in the NICU environment) compared to lying on their backs. Either way, she flipped him over and then took her arms out of the isolette's portholes and turned them over to me.

NICU nurses are notoriously and passionately protective of their babies, and I could feel the searing heat of her watchful eyes over my right shoulder. It's as close as I think I'll ever come to knowing what Frodo Baggins felt like with the Eye of Sauron bearing down on him and the Ring. I smiled and hesitatingly reached through the portholes into the warm and humid box holding the tiny creature now under my keep. At first, I couldn't actually see the baby. To protect premature babies' skin for the first several days after birth, the isolette's humidity is maintained at rainforest-like levels. In order to see inside the plastic panes, you have to wipe the dew off the interior surface with a washcloth. I did so, then examined the baby's head, heart, lungs, and belly. I reached my index finger toward his hand to check his perfusion and gently touched his palm. Even preemies have a fairly strong palmar grasp reflex, one that's deeply rooted in our mammalian evolutionary history from when newborns could grab onto their parents' body hair and go for a ride. He gripped my nail in a flash, wrapping fingers the size of Number 2 pencil lead around the nailbed of my index finger. I didn't know fingers that small were possible, and was surprised both by the strength and the speed that something so small could muster. After a moment, he let go, and having finished my exam I closed the doors to his isolette, and with an approving nod from the nurse I tossed my gloves, cleaned my hands, and moved on to my next patient.

It took that entire month during my intern block to really learn the unit's rules of engagement. Things like how to properly report a baby's urine output (milliliters per kilogram per hour), how a regular ventilator differs from a high-frequency ventilator, how to interpret a blood gas to know whether a ventilator is delivering too much, too little, or just the right amount of support to a baby's lungs, and, of course, what to do about all of it. I remember learning how to interact with new NICU parents, whose expressions ranged from deer-in-headlights shock to the bleary-eyed stare that said, "I've been up for 34 hours straight and will have no recollection of this conversation tomorrow." I also remember learning how to connect with "experienced" NICU parents, some of whom had been through many rounds of interns before me and knew way more about urine output, ventilator settings, and blood gases than any parent should ever have to learn.

That month I met babies born 16 weeks before their due dates and others born right on time but with massive congenital abnormalities. I cared for infants whose NICU stays were measured in hours alongside more than one who celebrated her first birthday in a NICU crib, having never left the hospital. Some were relatively well, requiring little treatment from us except time, some extra nutrition, or specialized light therapy for jaundice. Others were so sick we kept them medically paralyzed in a coma, on a high-frequency ventilator, with as many as eight intravenous pumps continuously delivering medications and fluids into their bodies and a pair of Bose noise-canceling headphones wrapped around their heads to make their worlds as still as possible.

As an intern, while I was the front-line, go-to doctor for all of these babies, I was surrounded by a team whose collective experience more than made up for my relative inexperience. I loved that sense of community—the

nurses, respiratory therapists, pharmacists, nurse practitioners, senior residents, fellows, and attendings who
all believed that the babies came first. When it became
clear that as an intern I felt the same way, I was quickly
brought "into the family."

Colleagues of mine didn't fare as well. Those who
don't come around to the NICU's way of thinking—
even if just for the four to six weeks interns spend there
during their first year—were excised like tumors. When
I returned to the NICU for my second and third tours
later in residency, these were the interns that I and the
rest of the team would encircle like hawks. Whereas
some residents were progressively allowed to do more,
treat younger and sicker babies, and advance their procedural skills during increasingly high-risk situations,
others were systematically maintained in as small and
safe a sandbox as possible. Glad to find myself in the
first batch, I was increasingly convinced that I should
pursue a career in neonatology.

Having long ago given up on adult cardiology, when
I started my pediatrics residency, I planned to specialize
in sports medicine and spend my life working as an outpatient pediatrician supporting high school, college, or
maybe even an Olympic sports team. During residency, though, I found myself drawn to two specialties that
were high-intensity, data-driven, and most heavily reli-
ant on strong communications skills—pediatric oncology and neonatology. On my pediatric oncology rotation, most of the kids were at least school age and could
engage in meaningful conversation, but they all faced
incredibly challenging cancer diagnoses and at best two
to three years of intense chemotherapy, radiation, and
sometimes surgery for a chance at long-term survival. I
was incredibly impressed that the treatment protocols

were very evidence-based, so much so that over 90% of children in America with the most common pediatric cancers are treated on some kind of active research protocol through the Children's Oncology Group[1]. However, pediatric oncology fellowship required participating in the kinds of basic science laboratory experiments that helped further the field but that I'd loathed during the summer I spent in Dr. Taplin's lab.

In neonatology, on the other hand, while the most premature infants faced extraordinarily long odds—23-weekers faced approximately 3 in 4 odds of death at the time I started fellowship—it felt like the entire NICU was both designed and driven to give them their absolute best chance at surviving and thriving. I remember as a second-year resident seeing the entire group of attending neonatologists descend upon the unit when one of their partners faced an especially challenging case. They huddled together near the main nurse's station like a football team facing fourth down and long, and emerged with a game plan that brought together the best of all their minds in a Borg-like collective intelligence. Every Monday the entire group also assembled in the large NICU conference room to review the previous week, discuss every patient who was admitted, any patient who died, and every patient who experienced some kind of setback. The team would also review the newest evidence published in medical journals to see if the NICU's protocols needed updating in some way to remain at the vanguard of the pediatric world.

Finally, and most attractive for me, each of the attending neonatologists had also become an expert not only in his or her clinical practice but in some other

---

1   https://www.childrensoncologygroup.org/

aspect of medicine or health care in general. One led clinical research for the department, one partnered with major analytics and industry groups to push the limits of quality improvement, one served as the Duke Health System's Chief Information Officer and still another co-founded the department's palliative care service. I wanted a career that would offer the same chance to be an outstanding clinician and a leader in some other aspect of medicine. Inspired by my time in the Duke NICU and all the people who served there, late in my second year of residency, I committed to pursuing three more years of dedicated NICU fellowship.

Almost as soon as I signed up, I suddenly found myself engaged in the toughest, most challenging cases in the unit. To make the leap into fellowship, I needed to up my game both intellectually and procedurally, so I took extra moonlighting calls as frequently as possible, spent holiday time in the NICU during the New Year's break and jumped in as backup for residents on family leave. Both the fellows and attending neonatologists brought me into their private conferences and shared the tricks they'd picked up through years and sometimes decades of practice. They also brought me into the NICU's clinical research teams, sparking an interest in quality improvement that would open new doors later in my career that at the time I couldn't have imagined. It was exciting, stimulating, motivating, and challenging, and I knew it was only a taste of what was to come.

My third year in residency had a few hard rotations but was largely elective-focused. During elective time, rotations without the service demands of every fourth or fifth night in-house call, I got more rest than I'd had in two years and would wind up having for another five. I also spent two weeks on the Special Care Nursery service at Durham Regional Hospital, a community hospital about 10 miles from Duke that I'd first visited as an intern and now returned to as a senior resident.

I loved Durham Regional (now called Duke Regional). While it had its own large delivery service, meaning we got to attend deliveries and occasionally had to resuscitate babies in the delivery room, the unit transferred out the sickest infants within hours of birth and transferred in babies from the main Duke NICU once they were stable "feeder growers." "Feeder grower" is a nickname for former preemies who, having made it through the highest-risk period of their NICU stay, really just need to grow and learn how to eat by mouth without using a supplemental feeding tube before they get to go home. The generally low-acuity census also allowed ample time to get to know the babies and their families, to read and learn, and to practice procedures on the simulation babies that the attendings kept in their office.

That particular month, though, we did admit one incredibly challenging baby, an infant whose story was rare at the time but would become increasingly common throughout my fellowship and into life as an attending today. His name was Noah* and he was born to a mother addicted to a smorgasbord of legal and illegal drugs that over the course of her pregnancy traversed through her bloodstream and into his. Infants like Noah were fairly uncommon in 2010 when I was a third-year resident. However, in Asheville, where I practice today, infants born exposed to maternal substance abuse account for up to 10% of the NICU's census at any given time and up to half of the babies I see in a typical morning at our NICU follow-up clinic. Opiate addiction is a scourge America has only just begun to address, but in

2010 most of the nation had yet to wake up to its damaging impact on both pregnancy and infancy.

Noah was a newborn when I first met him during my weeks on-service as a senior resident at Durham Regional, but I would come back to see him again and again over the coming months while taking weekend shifts and moonlighting calls. Today with close support from the Department of Social Services, NICUs are often able to discharge infants born with substance dependencies home to complete a gradual medication wean under the watchful eyes of their biological or foster parents, a community pediatrician, a social worker, and home health nurses. Noah was not one of those babies. Instead, both the severity of his withdrawal and his challenging social situation at home meant he had to stay in the Durham Regional Special Care Nursery to complete his baby version of a detoxification protocol.

Newborn Abstinence Syndrome, or NAS, can be a very, very serious condition. Some infants experience such severe withdrawal from whatever combination of drugs and/or prescribed medications their mothers were taking that they can experience seizures, coma, and even death. Importantly, these babies are not "born addicted." As Dr. Stephen Patrick, an old friend of mine from medical school and one of the nation's leading NAS researchers and advocates, notes, "It may seem like semantics, but that language fosters stigma. Babies cannot have an addiction by definition, because they cannot have inability to consistently abstain." Newborns are the involuntary recipients of whatever their mothers transferred to them through their shared placenta, whether legal or illegal. When that substance is a narcotic that leads to withdrawal and NAS, their cries can be piercing, their muscles tighter than a tick, and their agony so complete it can be exceptionally challenging even to feed a baby in the throes of true withdrawal.

Infants with NAS can be treated with a combination of both medication and non-medication-based therapies. In some of the mildest cases of withdrawal, infants don't need medications at all and respond to a quiet environment, undisturbed sleep, changes in feeding habits, and lots of rocking and skin-to-skin "kangaroo" care. Time is on your side when treating withdrawal, and often these non-pharmacologic interventions alone can bridge the baby long enough that the chemical dependency he was born with wears off. For others, the dependency is severe enough that babies need tiny doses of one or more medications like the ones their mothers had transferred to them through the placenta—drugs like methadone, morphine, and phenobarbital.

When treating NAS with medications like these, neonatologists start small and increase the doses gradually until we "capture" the baby's withdrawal symptoms. Capture may seem like a strange choice of verb, but trying to perfectly match a baby's withdrawal symptoms with just the right kind, amount, and timing of medication can feel like trying catch lightning bugs with your bare hands. Too aggressive an effort and you risk over-correcting, smashing the bug or sedating the baby —too meager an effort and you miss your chance entirely.

More challenging still, one of the most commonly used NAS medications–methadone–takes at least three doses (one given every 8-12 hours) to reach its "steady state" effect. Unlike a drug like fentanyl, a very powerful and very quick acting narcotic most often used to treat acute pain in the emergency department or the operating room, methadone is very slow acting and at "steady state" maintains a fairly steady concentration of narcotic in the bloodstream. This even-keeled balance can be great for treating NAS, but it means effectiveness of your attempt to "capture" the baby's symptoms can often more than a day to be able to assess and adjust. Only once finally captured, can we then start the very, very slow process of weaning the medications back off.

While my oldest daughter was not born with NAS, she had terrible colic. Colic is a condition that makes babies cry for no apparent reason—they're not hungry, they're not tired, and they don't need a diaper change; they just cry for hours at a time. When I started internship and a mother would tell me her baby had symptoms of colic, I'd talk through various possible treatment options and encourage her to sleep whenever she could. After Reese was born and we lived through the reality of colic in person, any time a mother told me her baby had colic symptoms I'd just break down, give her a hug, and tell her it wasn't her fault and that if she could just maintain her sanity for a few more weeks, everything was going to be OK.

Like babies with NAS, babies with colic sometimes respond to just rocking with them over and over and over again. Thus, Reese's infancy taught me to become an exceptionally skilled rocker, cuddler, and overall baby soother. As a result, when rounds would end at Durham Regional and Noah would still be screaming after his feeding, his medications, and a diaper change, I would put on a gown, pick him up, sit back in the rocking chair and rock. I would rock, and rock, and rock, and rock, until finally he'd go to sleep. We would stay like that, still together in the chair, until my pager beckoned me to leave.

More than once, just sitting down and rocking with

him wouldn't work and I had to break out my soon-to-be patented, maximum-strength baby soothing rocking method. I'd developed this method when Reese was at the peak of her colic symptoms and we couldn't even begin the process of sitting down with her even after she'd fallen asleep for fear of re-awakening the beast.

I'd start by standing and holding her cross-armed like I was cradling a football. Then I'd start bouncing my knees at a rate of about 120 bounces per minute, close to the resting heart-rate of a newborn and moving only a few inches up and down and up and down. When that failed, I'd move to level two and add in the back pat—with a hand that stretches from the top of a newborn's back to the mid-diaper, I've found a rate of about 360 pats a minute to be most effective in settling down a screaming newborn. Why 360 pats per minutes is the best rate I have no idea, but it works out to about three pats per knee bounce and sets up a nice rhythm as your body really begins to get into it in earnest. Level three requires adding a twist—which I do not recommend for anyone who's torn their ACL or had any other kind of knee surgery, because you need to twist from left to right or right to left with each knee bounce, mimicking the gentle back-and-forth rocking that an infant experiences inside the zero-gravity environment of a mother's amniotic-fluid-filled uterus.

The final level, which gets you to maximum-strength baby soothing power, involves either "hushing" out loud in time with the patting, twisting, or rocking, or singing whatever songs you've begun associating with the newborn's naptime. Since we'd only had one of our three children by this point, my personal song repertoire was fairly limited—with Reese I always started with "Somewhere Over the Rainbow," pivoted into "What a Wonderful World" and ended with a lilting rendition of "Rainbow Connection" in my best Kermit the Frog voice. If those three songs failed, I'd run through anything I could remember the words to, including songs by Green Day, Goo Goo Dolls, and I'm fairly sure the occasional Boyz II Men. I spared the Durham Regional Special Care Nursery the latter songbook, but figured if the first three were good enough for my own daughter, they'd be good enough for Noah. They generally were, and once he was asleep, I'd reverse the process by first stopping the singing, then the twisting, then the patting, and finally I'd excruciatingly slowly begin sitting down in a rocking chair to keep the rocking going off my feet.

It took the Special Care Nursery team weeks to find the right combination of drugs, doses, and human soothers to control Noah's withdrawal symptoms, and then months of gradually decreasing some component of the cocktail until they were all completely off for good. As a result, while Noah had just arrived as a newborn at Durham Regional when I first rotated through in the summer, he was still there cutting teeth and rolling over in his crib when I returned in the fall. I spent a weekend at Durham Regional just before Christmas and he was learning how to sit in a Bumbo chair and getting ready to begin eating baby foods. He was finally discharged home just before the spring thaw and not long before he learned how to crawl. All in all, Noah called the Durham Regional Hospital Special Care Nursery home for over six months, longer than any other baby anyone could remember and a tragic and 100% preventable way to spend one's infancy.

Bounding off successful months as a senior resident on the wards, in the clinics, and in the main Duke

– 3 –

Stand Tall on the Quarterdeck

"Hey!
I'm not giving up today,
There's nothing getting in my way,
And if you knock knock me over,
I will get back up again.
If something goes a little wrong,
Well you can go ahead and bring it on,
'Cause if you knock knock me over, I will get back up again."

–Poppy: *Trolls*

To really understand what NICU fellowship was like for me, there's a scene in the Russell Crowe movie *Master and Commander: The Far Side of the World* that, even if 19th century Napoleonic naval war battles aren't your thing, you need to see. Imagine the intrepid Captain Jack Aubrey, played by Crowe, finding his prey, the French privateer *Acheron*, at sea. As he closes his spyglass, the two tall ships engage in a fiery gun battle. The crew of his own imposing ship, the *HMS Surprise*, all take cover as French cannonballs pierce the sails, hull, and more than one of the *Surprise's* sailors. With the first volley over, Captain Aubrey paces the decks snapping orders to passing officers as the ship prepares its counterattack. Rounding the bend off the starboard beam, he comes upon the 13-year-old midshipman Lord Blakeney looking positively shell-shocked and still hunkered behind a rampart. Without pausing his stride, Aubrey reaches with his powerful arm, yanks the panic-stricken boy up by the collar, and says "We stand tall on the quarter-deck, son. All of us."

This scene was a favorite of my fellowship director and Duke's Chief of Neonatology Dr. Ronald Goldberg. Dr. Goldberg spent hours with me when I was a resident helping me work through what to do with my career, and his mentorship had a profound influence on my decision to commit to NICU fellowship. After I signed on during my second year of residency, he continued checking in with me from time to time and we ultimately began meeting every few months after I started my fellowship in July 2011. It was during one of those meetings that he first quoted the scene to me, sharing a concern first implicitly and then gradually more explicitly that—in no uncertain terms—if I wanted to succeed as a NICU fellow (and ultimately as any kind of leader) that I needed to stand taller.

Practicing medicine requires balancing many tensions—the tension between life and death, of healing and harming, of paternalism and partnership. Even the most successful doctors must also balance inside their own minds the tension between confidence and humility. I imagine the two like muses, something like the little angel and the little devil that sit on cartoon characters' shoulders as they debate the merits of their next zany antic. On the one side sits Confidence, bolstering a doctor's ego and whispering in his ear that he is an unstoppable force of clinical prowess and no one else in the world should be doing this thing (whatever it is) at this time other than him. On the other sits Humility, who serves a soft but firm reminder that—despite his delusions of grandeur—in reality a doctor is only human and therefore fallible. No one (but for perhaps cartoon characters), after all, is actually bulletproof.

Over the course of a career, the power balance between these seraphim in any doctor's mind waxes and wanes. At times, confidence overcomes the fear inherent to learning the practice of medicine, which—by design—requires practicing with other people's lives. At other times, humility restrains us from making potentially catastrophic mistakes of hubris when our skills clearly do not yet match the situation's demand. Each muse is necessary but insufficient both to individually practice medicine and for doctors collectively to advance the field. Without humility we would never have admitted bloodletting was (most often) a bad idea, and yet without an extreme level of confidence no human would have ever tried, much less perfected, the modern medical and surgical techniques that we take for granted today.

Take for example Dr. Michael E. Debakey, the first surgeon to successfully repair a rapidly expanding tear in the body's major central blood vessel called a thoracic aortic aneurysm. It's a daring surgery to say the least, involving burrowing into the core of a man's chest to keep the inside and outside walls of the aorta from tearing apart. Dr. DeBakey once told *Esquire* magazine, "It's important for a patient to go into an operation with confidence... the operation I did in '53 for aneurysm of the thoracic aorta gave me great satisfaction. It had never been done successfully before, and lots of doctors took the position that you shouldn't try it. You've got to push ahead in spite of them."

While I'm not a surgeon, I am certain it takes some serious steel nerves to walk into an operating room and believe that you and only you can save a person's life when all other surgeons have either failed or refused to even try. It was the kind of steel I knew I had inside me, confirmed through repeated victories over challenging clinical situations in both medical school and residency, yet had begun to elude me through those first few months of NICU fellowship. Even more precariously, in its place, humility had ballooned into full-blown fear.

When I started fellowship in the summer of 2011, I thought I was ready to handle the stress, responsibility, and degree of total chaos involved in running Duke's 68-bed Level IV NICU. On my first day of service, the off-going fellow handed me an emergency delivery pager, the "fellow phone," which every Labor and Delivery unit and hospital nursery in North Carolina had direct access to call, and gave me a half-hearted slap on the back. During daytime hours we had an army of people in the NICU, including nine large teams rounding on the babies, managing admissions, discharges, and transfers, and taking on the inevitable emergencies that arose in caring for so many critically ill patients at once. Overnight, however, the army scaled back to a small expeditionary force. At the time, Duke's NICU attendings took calls from home, leaving just the fellow, a resident, and generally two neonatal nurse practitioners in-house to cover the entire service. During residency I'd covered the similarly sized entire general pediatrics service and spent many nights on-call covering the NICU's resident teams, but I was in no way ready for the onslaught of decisions that hammered the in-house neonatology fellow 24 hours a day, seven days a week, and especially overnight.

For months I worked hard just to keep my head above the water line. After the daytime army left, I'd make it through every night (and there were a whole lot of nights) along with the rest of the unit. I called the attendings at home much more frequently than I imagine they intended, and constantly felt three steps too slow and markedly less shrewd than I needed to be to keep the NICU's lid from boiling over. Worse still, when it did boil over, I boiled over too, the stress evident in my face, my voice, and my demeanor in ways that impacted the morale of the entire NICU team. A fearful fellow does not inspire confidence.

I remember standing at the main NICU nurse's station on one particularly harrowing night in late February. I was staring at both the nastiest admission board and perhaps the angriest charge nurse I'd ever seen. I had just walked up to the board to tell her we simultaneously had one baby with blood sugar problems needing to come up for treatment from the full-term nursery, a mother in Labor and Delivery ready to deliver 28-week twins at any moment, and an outside hospital holding on the phone that desperately needed to transfer a baby with hypoxic ischemic encephalopathy to us for whole-body cooling. I hadn't been able to keep her updated as call after call poured into the fellow's phone and now I didn't know where to start. Standing cross-armed in front of the enormous whiteboard, her eyes bored into me with a stare that said "you need to tell me exactly what in God's name is going on RIGHT NOW."

You don't get to be a NICU charge nurse without first having developed a great deal of comfort in managing through chaos. Yet even the best charge nurses need a doctor—in this case the Duke NICU fellow—to help them navigate the waves of a stormy night shift. Charge nurses only have so many levers they can pull on their own—in this case, the very experienced charge nurse on that night knew she could shuffle assignments, call in extra nurses from home, and even temporarily take on a bedside patient assignment herself, all to temporize a unit that might wind up housing more babies than it had beds at least until the morning. But for her to do so and maintain the unit on some semblance of an even keel, she needed me to keep her continually informed on what was coming in, when it was coming, which babies could be discharged out and to where. The longer the lead time on all of this information the better, and I was about to dump it all on the table in one fell swoop. It was clear that I wasn't stepping up to the leadership test, and at that moment I felt as overwhelmed as I'd ever felt in my life.

The team that night, of course, pulled together as all great teams do. We briefly housed infants four to a room that usually fit only three, admitted the hypoglycemic baby from the well-baby nursery and brought his sugar up with intravenous dextrose, stabilized the 28-week twins on CPAP after their uneventful delivery, and even settled in the transfer baby on his therapeutic hypothermia protocol all before the day-time army bounded back through the doors at 7 a.m. Once again, both I and the NICU's throng of babies ultimately survived the night, but it was clear to both me and her that something needed to change. She found her way to Dr. Goldberg—an act of kindness I'm incredibly grateful for today—and he ultimately found his way to me.

Confidence can be a funny thing. For athletes who are "in the zone," a sense of confidence can become so overwhelming that baseball players sometimes describe 98 MPH major league fastballs as looking like beachballs floating to the plate in slow motion. Success generally breeds more success, and history is replete with examples of players whose confidence when "in the zone" spurred them on to career-defining streaks. While nowhere close to Joe DiMaggio's record 56 consecutive game hitting streak for the New York Yankees in 1941, I had a streak like this when I was a senior in high school playing for Algonquin Regional's baseball team. For reasons I'll never be able to explain, I started that season feeling incredibly confident and for the first 10 games of the year, I nearly led the league in both batting average and hits. I was on fire, hitting anything anywhere near the plate and hitting balls harder and farther than ever before (and ever since).

Yet sooner or later every streak breaks, and when it does, even the best player begins to question things. He questions his bat, his grip, his stance, his batting gloves, even his longstanding pre-at-bat rituals. Confidence shaken, he's back to the drawing board, left to wonder where "the magic" went. By the time Dr. Goldberg sat me in his expansive office on the fifth floor of the Hock Plaza building in March of 2012, I'd reached the same point in fellowship as I'd reached when my 10-game hitting streak came to a screeching halt back in high school. I questioned my intellectual skills as a doctor, I questioned my procedural skills as a pediatrician and neonatal intensivist, and I ultimately questioned the decision I'd made to enter NICU fellowship at all.

The doubts I felt were so deep that I strongly considered leaving the program, breaking away from medicine entirely, and going to work as a management consultant with an old colleague in Chicago. Instead, Dr. Goldberg handed me a strong cup of espresso, looked me square in the eyes, and told me to stand tall on the quarterdeck. He said I needed to believe in myself if I wanted anyone to believe in me, and that as a NICU fellow I needed the NICU staff to believe in me. He had built the Duke NICU to be a fellow-run unit, which meant while the attendings were the masterminds behind all important treatment trajectories, it was the fellow who took charge as the unit's leader. If the team of nurses, nurse practitioners, respiratory therapists, students, and residents was going to reach its peak performance—and we had to be at our best to give every one of our babies the best chance to triumph over adversity—I would need to step up and stand tall in a fundamentally different way.

Life brings all of us at least a handful of spectacularly ephemeral encounters with great triumph. They can be individual or team-based, personal or professional, very private or very public. By triumph I don't just mean "good" or happy experiences—I mean real victory in the face of long odds, a hard-fought battle that ends with right prevailing over wrong. It took one of these triumphs for me to finally turn the corner in my first year of NICU fellowship, involving treating an infant with a condition called persistent pulmonary hypertension (PPHN). Every victory against PPHN—a disease that has given me (and most neonatologists) more nightmares, heartburn, and gray hair than all others combined—is a small triumph, but to fully appreciate why, I need to tell you more about the condition itself.

When a baby is born, a miraculous combination of physiologic events happens that forces developmental fetal fluid out of the lungs and fills them instead with oxygen. The influx of oxygen opens wide the baby's pulmonary blood vessels, allowing the life-long exchange of oxygen and carbon dioxide to begin. With the rapid influx of oxygen, the baby's blood reddens and his skin quickly fills with the pinkish flush of life.

Recent evidence suggests that this nearly magical sequence of events happens normally in about 998 out of 1,000 births. The other 0.2% of the time something else happens, leaving the pulmonary blood vessels tightly constricted. Constricted blood vessels don't carry much blood, owing to the principle first described by 19th century French physiologist Jean Léonard Marie Poiseuille. He discovered a 4th-power exponential relationship between the radius of a blood vessel and the vessel's resistance to blood flow. In plain English, this means a blood vessel that is 1/4th its usual size will only have 1/64th its usual flow. A 64-fold change is equivalent to a 98.4% drop, or roughly the same as taking the entire Mississippi River at its widest point near Bena, Minnesota, and squeezing its corpulent 11-mile girth down into a channel the size of a high school running track.

This is a really important concept in neonatal pulmonary mechanics, because it means a small change in the size of a constricted pulmonary blood vessel has a very large impact on how much blood can actually flow through it. No blood flow means no exchanging oxygen for carbon dioxide, and no oxygen means a very blue baby. This is more or less what happens with PPHN.

Babies with PPHN often need to be intubated in the delivery room and wind up quickly needing 100% oxygen mixed with a special medication called nitric oxide that seems to help selectively dilate pulmonary blood vessels. Their first chest x-rays look like a car's windshield in the middle of a blizzard: total white-out. They have oxygenation problems, ventilation problems, agitation problems, and blood pressure problems, any one of which can send the baby's entire physiologic balance into a downward spiral. Treating PPHN must feel similar to the way carnival plate spinners feel once they get all 12 plates going at once—eyes and hands darting from plate to plate, knowing that if you lose the rhythm even for a second to save one plate, the rest will come crashing to the ground. Except for a baby with PPHN, losing that balance doesn't lead to broken chinaware— it leads to death.

Some of my greatest private triumphs in medicine have come at the bedside of babies with PPHN, including the one that followed soon after Dr. Goldberg's pep talk. On that particular call night, I wound up staying at a baby's bedside for what must have been 14 hours straight. His name was Alex*, and while I'd cared for several babies with PPHN over the first nine months of fellowship, he was without a doubt the sickest. Alex was born exceptionally ill—the delivery room team spent 45 minutes resuscitating him before his heart rate was high enough to stop CPR, and when he was admitted to the NICU, he was immediately placed on the therapeutic hypothermia protocol. Therapeutic hypothermia is a treatment used for newborns whose bodies and brains are temporarily deprived of oxygen, most often before or during the delivery process. Pioneering clinical trials in the early 2000s demonstrated that intentionally cooling babies whose symptoms are consistent with temporary oxygen deprivation down to 33 degrees Celsius for 72 hours improves their chances of avoiding severe neurologic and developmental issues.

I'd treated numerous infants with therapeutic hypothermia, but Alex's case was different because he also had profound PPHN. Managing PPHN is hard enough at a normal body temperature—it's nearly impossible when an already irritable baby is now both shivering and splenetic. I spent hour after hour with Alex, leveraging every aspect of my clinical brain to stay one step ahead of his disease. After five cups of coffee and hundreds of small adjustments, we finally "captured" him around midnight, reaching a state of relative stability in the midst of his critical illness on significantly high ventilator settings, ungodly doses of multiple blood pressure medications, and a cocktail of sedative and paralytic medications that kept him both relaxed and quiet. We even put a pair of noise-canceling headphones over his ears, knowing even the slightest disturbance to his restful state could restart the downward spiral we had spent so many hours to arrest.

Alex was the first newborn whose bedside I quite literally kept vigil over all night until the morning team arrived at 7 a.m. to take over the next watch. I remember sitting in a swivel chair, elbows resting on the nurses' table, chin resting on my knuckles. I watched the digital shimmers of his monitor screen like a hawk—the pulsatile wave of the blue pulse oximetry line, the regular and repetitive morphology of the green electrocardiogram line, the red continuous arterial blood pressure lines' nearly sinusoidal progression, and the sawtooth-like bounce of the yellow line intended to monitor respiratory rate but totally useless with a high-frequency ventilator vibrating the boy's chest eight times each second. Every few minutes we'd tweak some parameter ever so slightly, inching one of the blood pressure medications up just a hair or one of 15 different ventilator settings down a nudge, always trying to stay at least one step ahead of his disease and keep all the plates spinning.

In the grand scheme of things, keeping Alex alive until morning may have been a small triumph, but for him, his family, and for me, it was much more. Alex would ultimately survive his PPHN, spend several months in the NICU convalescing, and be discharged home with great fanfare later that year. For me, I finally felt like I could chalk up a real triumph, a baby I believed was meaningfully given a better chance at surviving because he had me on call as his NICU fellow that night. Not that any other doctor couldn't have gotten him through the battle, but I knew I had given him the fullest measure of my devotion and had come out on top. Success breeds success, and my victory that night against the dueling evils of PPHN and therapeutic hypothermia bolstered my confidence and righted the trajectory of my path as a neonatology fellow.

Some people are born able to stand tall and project a calm confidence in the face of mortal adversity. For the rest of us, I think we're born with the capacity to do so but only learn how through lived experience. During fellowship, I spent a lot of time learning to navigate the infinite corners of hyperspecialized NICU medicine. I read thousands of pages of textbooks and articles, attended hundreds of poster and platform presentations, and did more research than I'd done in all 30-plus previous years of my education combined. I honed my procedural skills, intubating baby after baby until the movements became rote muscle memory, and placed more umbilical lines than there were umbilici in my first-year medical school class. But more than the medical or procedural knowledge, in fellowship I learned both how to stand tall on the quarterdeck and how to communicate that confidence to others, especially to patients and their parents under the most extreme circumstances life has to offer.

Medicine is fundamentally about communication—

doctors communicating with nurses, doctors communicating with other doctors, teams communicating with teams, and ultimately everyone communicating with patients and their families. Medical school did a reasonable job of teaching me how to talk to other doctors, but it only scratched the surface on how to really connect and communicate with patients. We did have several class simulations on "delivering bad news" with an attending pediatric dermatologist named Dr. Neil Prose. At the time, I hated Dr. Prose's sessions because we'd role-play speaking with a patient (Dr. Prose) about a devastating diagnosis while we were recorded on video. We'd stumble through the session and then he'd sit with us and individually review our video.

I remember my videos being horrifically bad at first. I never remembered to "fire a warning shot" to alert the patient that I was about to communicate something really important. I never paused to allow the serious, life-changing news to sink in. What's worse, without fail I always rushed through the emotional part of each discussion to get to the logical, data-driven evidence I knew I needed to share in order to begin designing a treatment path. We practiced and practiced throughout medical school and into residency, yet despite Dr. Prose's best efforts I resigned myself to the fact that his lessons just wouldn't stick.

My first real opportunity to use these lessons in practice came later in residency while I was working in the pediatric emergency department. I was the most senior resident covering an evening shift, and the place was packed with a full waiting room of patients waiting to be seen. In a bit of a rush, I picked up the next electronic chart in the stack and went to see a child named "Anna*" in room 4 whose chief complaint was reportedly "constipation." Constipation isn't generally a real emergency department issue, so I figured we could "treat and street" her pretty quickly and I'd be able to move on to the next patient in the queue.

When I got to the room, I found an incredibly nervous but incredibly charming set of young parents and a child of no more than 12 months old. Anna was sitting unsettlingly still for a baby her age in her mother's lap and she looked downright mopey. I sat down next to her on the obligatory doctor's rolling stool, introduced myself, and asked them to tell me about Anna's constipation. They said Anna was having a really hard time having a bowel movement, that she'd had the problem now for weeks if not months, that they'd tried pear juice, prune juice, and every kind of over-the-counter laxative on the market, but none of it worked because her belly was always hard. As our discussion progressed, it became apparent that Anna's problems didn't stop at constipation. Her parents noticed that her developmental progress had also stalled—she couldn't crawl, couldn't sit, and could barely roll over, all skills we expect most children to have mastered this late into their first year of life.

By the time I washed my hands to perform a physical exam, I knew that this would not be a quick "treat and street" emergency department visit for constipation. I was terribly nervous about what I'd find when I mashed on Anna's belly, so of course I performed literally every other aspect of a complete textbook physical exam first. I listened to her heart and lungs, checked her reflexes, thoroughly assessed the function of each of her 12 cranial nerves individually, and evaluated the perfusion in her hands and feet, all of which were essentially fine. Unable to avoid it further, I then softly pushed on her abdomen.

In kids Anna's age, bellies are usually as soft as a couch pillow unless the child is laughing or crying. She was doing neither, just staring at me with a belly as hard as a rock and a softball-sized mass right in the middle. I took a deep breath, told her parents I was as concerned as they were about her belly and her frozen developmental progress and that I was grateful they brought her to the emergency department that night. I said we would need to run some bloodwork and get a CT scan and I'd be back to talk again as soon as we had some results.

Two hours later I was sitting in an incredibly uncomfortable chair staring at an incredibly bright computer screen. Anna had just returned from her CT scan, and having pulled up the images, I saw staring back at me both exactly what I'd anticipated and exactly what I desperately hoped wouldn't be there—a cantaloupe-sized tumor, nestled in the middle of her body just in front of her thoracic spine. I poked the arm of my attending physician seated at the next computer over and said, "Look at this CT scan—I was right, this child must have cancer." He agreed, and then asked me when I was going to tell them. My jaw nearly hit the keyboard. While we couldn't be positive without a biopsy, telling parents their kid very likely has cancer seemed like the kind of thing a resident didn't (or at least shouldn't) get to do. But the emergency department was busy, and the attending was juggling multiple critical patients himself. "You've got this," he said, resting a hand on my shoulder, "just be patient, speak from your heart, and you'll be fine. Oh, and remember to fire a warning shot."

The assignment clear, I took several minutes to myself preparing for the conversation that would come next. I made a lap around the emergency department's private exterior corridor, rehearsing what I'd say and how I'd say it, trying to be compassionate while projecting the confidence needed to help young parents step through an abyss and back on the path to healing. All the while recognizing that immediately after hearing the word "cancer" their eyes would glaze, their world would turn sideways, and I might as well be reading aloud from a Cantonese translation of the *Declaration of Independence*.

It was during those few minutes of solitude in the back hallway of the Duke pediatric emergency department that I realized for the first time I was about to divide someone's life in half. The first half was everything Anna's mother and father had experienced up to that moment—the second would be everything that happened after they learned that their baby had cancer. While it wasn't my fault their baby had cancer, it would be my fault if all they remembered about that awful night was how awful the doctor was who told them their baby had cancer. It's the kind of thing I really, really didn't want to screw up, and the kind of thing I was now grateful I'd practiced so many times with Dr. Prose.

I remember walking up to Anna's room, taking a deep breath, and knocking on the glass window. When her parents opened the door, I sat again on the rolling stool, logged in to the computer attached to the wall, and said we needed to talk about Anna's results. I can't remember any of the specific words I used, but without question I followed Dr. Prose's recipe to the letter. I first fired the warning shot, telling the parents we had some very difficult news we needed to discuss. Then I paused, pulled up the CT scan images, and showed them the mass. As the three of us looked at the monster glowing back at us in black and white from the computer screen, I said something to the effect of, "I can't be sure of it until we get a biopsy, but in all likelihood, Anna has cancer."

At that moment I quite literally bit my tongue hard enough it almost started to bleed and I silently counted to seven. Psychologists note that most Americans can tolerate anywhere from five to seven seconds of total silence before speaking up just to break the quiet—under these circumstances, without intense focus my brain could tolerate perhaps five to seven microseconds. I badly wanted to tell them how we'd formulate a battle plan, admit her to the hospital, perform the biopsy, diagnose the cancer, and identify our enemy down to its most microscopic molecular signature. We'd then send her to surgery to remove the tumor and get her on the best, most up-to-date and evidence-based chemotherapy protocol in the world for whatever leviathan she had growing astride her spine.

That night, however, I'd finally understood that none of what I wanted to share was what they actually needed to hear. Right then, more than anything else, they needed silence. They needed time to process, time to recognize that the gravitational field maintaining order within the galaxy of their lives had just reversed polarity and it would be awhile before they could think about getting the stars, planets, and moons back into orbit. So instead of launching into a dissertation on everything I knew about aggressively battling pediatric cancer, I sat with them in silence as the magnitude of their new reality gradually set in.

After what felt like an eternity, their eyes unglazed and they asked a few questions. I answered them all, then said I would step out to give them a few minutes alone with Anna and to call our oncology team. I had worked with each of the pediatric oncology doctors personally, including the one on call that night, and said they were all caring, bright, and dedicated people who would spend as much time as we needed to talk through the immediate next steps. Finally, before I left the room, I said I would be there for them and with them all night, no matter what, to talk through anything at any time as many times as they needed. Then I rose from the rolling stool, opened the door, walked back to the emergency department physician's workstation, and cried.

While my career path took me away from pediatric cancer and into the NICU instead, the conversation with Anna's parents turned out to be only the first of many discussions of life and death I'd face in practice. For me, the hardest of these "life dividing" discussions take place in Labor and Delivery rooms with expecting mothers (and their families) who go into labor before medicine gives us the ability to even try to resuscitate their babies. I've walked with parents through every possible emotion during conversations like these, and each family's circumstances are different. Some expectant mothers have been in the hospital for weeks, having had their water break very early in pregnancy and been admitted to a maternal-fetal medicine unit for bed-rest, antibiotics, and more than anything else, hope. Hope that both mother and baby will stay well enough long enough to give the unborn baby a chance at survival. For others, the entire pregnancy has been normal right up until the day they arrive at the hospital when, all of a sudden, it's not. And while I remember every single one of these conversations, there is one family I remember today as vividly as the day I met them.

I met them on a weekend late in my NICU fellowship when I was the only NICU fellow in the unit. The fellow phone rang and I saw the number to Labor and Delivery pop up on the Caller ID. My pulse quickened—Labor and Delivery rarely called the fellow's phone directly and when they did it was never good news. When I answered I found one of the OB-GYN residents on the other end of the line, and she asked me to come to their workroom. I said I would, and since we couldn't hear the NICU's dedicated "code bell" outside of the unit, I let the resident, neonatal nurse practitioners, and the NICU charge nurse know I was heading over to Labor and Delivery.

I crossed the threshold of the NICU's double doors, entered Labor and Delivery, and sat down at the large table in the OB-GYN workroom surrounded by the same anatomic models that a different generation of OB-GYN residents used to teach me how to guide a baby's head through the birth canal as a medical student. The OB-GYN resident stood up from her computer and joined me at the table. As a NICU fellow, you quickly learn to differentiate between the OB-GYN residents who call you often and those who don't—this doctor fell into the latter category. We knew each other well from many nights and weekends spent in the hospital together but on opposite sides of the birthing spectrum, and I knew if she was asking me for help, she really needed it.

She got right to it. "Chris, you know I don't normally call you for this, but I need to you to talk to a mother who's having a miscarriage."

"Sure," I said, "can you tell me more?"

"They're a young family and the mom-to-be is in labor and has chorio. She's getting sick and we have to deliver her, but she's only 21 weeks pregnant and I've spent the last hour talking them through why we can't try to save the baby. I've tried everything I know and it's not helping. I thought maybe coming directly from you it might be easier to accept."

Chorio is short for chorioamnionitis, a dangerous and rapidly progressing infection inside the uterus of a pregnant woman that left untreated can lead to death. Antibiotics are sometimes helpful very early in the course, but the only definitive treatment involves both antibiotics and delivery so the uterus can begin clearing the infection without a placenta, amniotic sac, and a baby inside it. Chorioamnionitis is also incredibly dangerous for babies, as the infection can work its way through the placenta and into the baby's bloodstream. Bacteria in a baby's bloodstream rapidly leads to sepsis (also sometimes called "blood poisoning"), shock, and death. It's nothing to trifle with.

I knew that the OB-GYN resident was boxed into a corner, a corner she had talked through with all of her colleagues, her attending physician, and the maternal-fetal medicine specialists who served only the sickest and highest-risk pregnancies. The mother's labor meant the baby was coming now, and while delivery meant certain death for the infant, stalling labor with medications in a desperate attempt to continue the pregnancy still likely meant death for the baby and a very high risk of death for the mother. They were as certain as OB-GYNs could be about the dating of the pregnancy, which given that it fell on the wrong side of the limit of viability made it an impossibly hard recommendation. It was, however, unequivocally the right one.

I thanked her for sharing the full details of the patient's story and opened the electronic medical record myself so I could review everything and learn even more about the mother and her husband. They were indeed young, both in their early 20s, recently married, and both beginning professional careers. I'd been told by the resident that several of the parents' family members including both sets of their parents would be in the room waiting when I went to see them and to be ready for lots, and lots, and lots of questions.

Following a variation on the *House of God's* Third Law, I took a deep breath and checked my own pulse before heading into the room. I'd come a long way since Anna by this point in fellowship, and had had lots of hard conversations with parents. Even though I hadn't met this exact family under these exact circumstances before, I knew I'd be ready. I took a few deep breaths, forced my heart rate down from the mid 90s to the high 60s, knocked on the door, and entered the room. I introduced myself first to the mother and father-to-be, then to the dozen or so family members encircling the bed, the couch, and every other piece of furniture crammed into the birthing suite. Then I pulled up the ever-present doctor's rolling stool and we started to talk. I asked the patient and her husband to tell me what they understood about what was happening—the unborn baby's father spoke up and talked about the labor, the infection, and the need to not stop the labor because of the seriousness of the infection. I told them they had it right, that trying to stop the labor now wasn't going to lead to a different outcome for their baby, but it had great risk of leading to a very different outcome for the mother, and that I agreed with the OB-GYN team's recommendation.

We talked for what must have been nearly an hour about the kinds of things we normally try to save a premature baby's life, and about why, at the time, NICUs would not begin resuscitating a baby born at 21 weeks but would at 23 weeks. If you remember no other clinical facts about NICU medicine from this book, I hope you'll remember that a single week matters more in pregnancy and prematurity than at any other time in a human's life.

As the conversation drew to a close, the patient's husband looked up at me. His hands were clasped so tightly his knuckles were as white as the sheet on his wife's bed. He wasn't that much younger than me, but he was much more muscular, and I could see the veins in his forearms bulging as he wrung his hands together like the springs of a catapult. His eyes were red and tearful as he looked up and said, "Doctor, is there really nothing, not a single thing that you can do to save my daughter?"

This stopped me cold. I was already a father in my own right well before I started NICU fellowship, and being a father has fundamentally shaped the way I communicate with parents. While I am more than confident that pediatricians without children are incredible communicators, I've found that having three children of my own gives me an emotional lane to connect with parents on a very personal level, and in conversations like these I don't try to hide my emotion.

His words knocked me momentarily off beat. I thought about my kids, about what I would do to save their lives. I could feel the combination of anger and sadness in his voice. I could see it in his hands. My own hands were physically trembling and I've never fought harder to hold back tears. It didn't work. My eyes filled with tears, my voice ever so slightly wavered, and I brought my gaze to meet his. I then said, "It is my job to bring all that medicine has to bear to save babies. If there was literally anything that I and the massive team of NICU caregivers behind me could possibly do, I would do it. But I can't. And I am infinitely sorry."

There are few things more humbling than admitting you are powerless to change something, and that moment was without exception the most humbling experience of my life.

Confidence and humility, strength and compassion, success and failure—I'd find them all in more or less equal measure over three years of NICU fellowship. From moments when the world humbled me in ways I'd never envisioned possible, to moments like the night I spent with Alex holding back the enemy at the gates, fellowship taught me when to stand tall and how best to play my part in the constant tension between life and death.

– 4 –

Alpha and Omega

"After all, what's a life, anyway? We're born, we live a little
while, we die. A spider's life can't help being something of a
mess, with all this trapping and eating flies. By helping you,
perhaps I was trying to lift up my life a trifle. Heaven knows
anyone's life can stand a little of that."

–Charlotte: *Charlotte's Web*

In modern life, it's increasingly rare for most people
to encounter either life's Alpha or Omega—birth and
death—with any meaningful frequency. Take my father—he's 61 years old and has spent his entire professional life in engineering and construction. He's been
close to exactly three births—mine, my sister's, and my
brother's—though all three of us were born well before
the concept of really engaging fathers in the Labor and
Delivery suite had become commonplace. And having
been born a few years too late to have been drafted and
shipped to Vietnam, he's been close to exactly one death.
It happened on a jobsite when he was in his 20s, when a

cylinder exploded through the chest of one of the men he worked with and left a gaping, cauterized hole in his thorax before the man's body crumpled to the ground.

My experience as a doctor has been much different, as during fellowship my professional world began frequently intersecting the orbits of both birth and death. While for many people these two core human experiences seem somehow foreign, I can promise you that they're not. Though the newness of taking part in either wears off over time, the uniquely human aspect of each experience is hard to describe.

My first experience with death actually happened before I even went to medical school. It was 18 years ago, when I was a 19-year-old emergency department (ED) technician in Worcester, Massachusetts. I'd earned my Emergency Medical Technician (EMT) license as a freshman in college, and that summer got a job working in the local hospital's ED. I took the job in part because it paid better than working as an EMT on an ambulance, and because I got to do things like electrocardiograms and blood draws that EMTs weren't allowed to do in the field.

I'd been working in the ED for a few weeks in the summer of 2001 when an ambulance brought an elderly patient through the trauma bay's double doors in full cardiac arrest. Her heart had stopped, she collapsed, her family called 911, and now we had to try to save her. As an ED technician I couldn't start an IV, I couldn't give any drugs, and I wasn't allowed to implement the Advanced Cardiac Life Support protocol that everyone else in the room had trained, drilled, and practiced repeatedly. But I was an EMT and I did know how to do CPR, though at that point, despite compressing the chests of more mannequins than I could count, I'd never actually done it on a person.

My role now clear, after we transferred the woman from the ambulance's stretcher into the ED bed, I climbed up a small step-stool, grasped the knuckles of my left hand with the palm of my right hand, and began giving a real patient CPR for the first time as the entire ED team tried to save her life. We didn't. After 20 minutes of resuscitation, during which I learned exactly how hard it really is to give good quality chest compressions to an actual adult human, the ED physician called the code and declared her dead. I was drenched in sweat and physically exhausted... and had no idea what happened next.

As it turned out, my job as an ED technician also involved helping prepare the elderly woman's frail body after death for the morgue. We cleaned the blood from her IV sticks, changed her sheets, dimmed the lights, and welcomed a full cast of family and friends into the trauma bay. They stayed with her in the softly lit room for hours. When late in my shift they said their last goodbyes, a more experienced ED technician and I returned to make the final preparations to transfer her "downstairs." I remember being surprised at how quickly the warmth had drained from her body when we moved the sheet to fasten a body tag to her toe, supplementing the ID band around her wrist. We then used the bottom sheet to move her body onto the box-like morgue stretcher, draping yet another clean white sheet over its top rails and thus hiding the shape of her body from passersby in the hospital halls.

Ready now for our trip, the other ED technician led the way to the elevator and down to the morgue. Once inside, we opened a small door the size of a college dorm-room refrigerator, pulled out a metal slide, transferred her body, and pushed the slide back in. We then closed the door and affixed another label to the door's outer tag slot. That was it. We left the morgue, washed our hands, walked back upstairs, and went back to work. I have no recollection whatsoever of what happened for the rest of my shift, but will never forget the woman, her family, the morgue, or the tag.

My first experience with birth (not counting my own) was 13 years ago, when I was a 24-year-old medical student in Durham, North Carolina. I was a little over halfway through my second year of medical school, the year that Duke medical students rotated through all the basic medical and surgical specialties and mere weeks before I'd meet my wife in that fateful second-floor lecture hall. It was springtime and I was excited to start my rotation on Labor and Delivery because medical students on Labor and Delivery got to deliver babies. Not stand to the side while the real doctors delivered babies—I mean actually deliver a baby with our own two hands.

The day arrived and I remember cleaning my hands with the betadine scrub brush, gowning and gloving just like I'd learned on my surgery clerkship, and sitting on the metal stool at the foot of the soon-to-be mother's bed with the dutiful resident physician hovering over my left shoulder. It wasn't this mother's first baby and we expected her to deliver pretty quickly.

The mother-to-be was already in the stirrups of the specialized Labor and Delivery bed ready to push, and by the time I was in position the baby's head was already crowning. The resident coached me through carefully delivering the baby's head, checking to ensure his umbilical cord hadn't slipped around his neck and making sure the shoulders didn't follow too quickly. There's sort of a "pop" when a baby's head completely delivers that I remember seemed somewhat shocking, but the resident didn't look worried so I made sure to hide the surprise from my face as well.

With the baby's head safely delivered, the resident talked me through how to gently tilt the soon-to-be newborn's body just right so we could deliver one shoulder and then the next. That's when I realized exactly how slippery a newborn baby can be. His first shoulder delivered just as expected, but then his second shoulder emerged with a speed and force I hadn't appreciated was possible during childbirth and the rest of his body quickly followed suit. I managed to catch his tiny butt with my right hand while the resident's arms flashed with lightning speed and flipped the rest of his body up onto my left forearm and into a stable position.

Pound for pound, at that moment my adrenaline level and the newborn's adrenaline level must have been about equal, as the fact that I almost just dropped a baby sank in. Thanks only to a quick hand (all that baseball I played as a kid had finally paid off), a superbly mindful resident, and a whole lot of luck, I didn't. And now this new little person was alive, and screaming, and pooping right in my hands. I handed him to his mother and she smiled, his slippery little body now nuzzled against hers in much the same way he had been nuzzled against her insides for the last nine months.

I delivered at least one more baby on that 24-hour shift and assisted with several more over the course of my rotation on Labor and Delivery, but this first experience with birth has stayed with me. The look on his mother's face when she held him, the intense fear of almost dropping a baby as slippery as a greased pig, the hands of the resident imperceptibly hovering then shooting forward at just the right moment, and the silent reassurance I gave myself that the resident's deftness must have been a sign that it wasn't the first time she'd had to help a hapless medical student not drop a newborn.

As a doctor who works with very sick and premature infants, I have now been present for many, many more births and many more deaths since these first experiences. While I've mercifully never had to deliver another baby since medical school—though I got very, very close to having to deliver my own son near the end of fellowship—my work in neonatology has brought me to the bedside to care for hundreds of newborns at the time of their births. In general, neonatologists aren't called to the delivery for "normal" births, so my time in delivery rooms in the decade since I finished medical school have come with the very real possibility of simultaneously experiencing both birth and death.

When you're called to a delivery to care for the newborn, you can learn a lot about what to expect in just the text of the page that calls you there. As an intern in pediatric residency, we began carrying "delivery pagers" that would go off whenever an OB-GYN team anticipated they may need help. Sometimes the page would just give a room number like "DR team to 5407." DR stood for "delivery room" and it generally meant the OB-GYNs anticipated a delivery with a fairly low risk of problems. An intern and a second-year resident usually answered those pages along with an experienced NICU nurse and a respiratory therapist, but most of the time the baby would have been just fine if no one showed up. I went to nearly a hundred such deliveries during my intern year, and rarely had to do more than dry off the screaming babies with a towel and suck out their noses with one of those blue bulb suction devices (which invariably made them scream more). We'd keep these babies at the warmer bed long enough to assign the mandatory one-minute and five-minute APGAR scores, which is a 0-10 rating system developed by Dr. Virginia Apgar that more or less objectively tells how well a baby is transitioning to post-uterine life. Then we'd pop on a diaper, an ID band, and a hat, swaddle the baby up, and hand either him or her back to a now smiling mother. I got very, very good at swaddling.

Sometimes the page was more urgent, like "STAT to 5407." The "STAT" pages usually increased the speed with which the team answering the call ran down the hallway and generally brought the whole regular delivery team plus one or more senior providers. After finishing three years of pediatric residency and starting NICU fellowship, these were the kind of pages I now responded to along with the intern, the resident, the nurse, and the respiratory therapist. While most of the babies at these deliveries ultimately did fine, some actually needed basic resuscitation beyond warming, drying, and stimulating them to breathe. This usually involved giving rescue breaths, where you use a small hand-powered AMBU bag or gas-powered T-piece respirator with a mask and blow oxygen mixed with air into the baby's lungs to kick-start their crying. It's amazing how quickly babies who initially look a little purple can pink right up after one or two rounds of positive pressure ventilation, and as long as they turned the corner within a few minutes, they too would get diapered, banded, swaddled, and handed off to their slightly more nervous but still smiling parents.

The most concerning pages would just read "OB EMER 5407." I never figured out if there wasn't enough space on the pager to fit the full text of "OB EMER-GENCY" or if whoever was typing never felt like they had enough time to do so. Either way it was clear what it meant, and an "OB EMER" page would get half the NICU up and running toward the Labor and Delivery suites. Even late in fellowship, these were the pages that got my heart rate up because they meant we would likely need to draw on our most specialized NICU skill-sets to save a very high-risk newborn's life.

If you look at broad population-level measures, about 1 in 10 newborns will need some degree of support in the delivery room, ranging from vigorous stimulation to a few minutes of positive pressure ventilation. Less than 1 in 10 of those babies (or less than 1% of all newborns) will need more serious help including more aggressive or extended positive pressure ventilation with higher concentration oxygen, intubation with a breathing tube, CPR, emergency medications, blood, or fluid.

When you're running down the hallway for a page that reads "OB EMER," with a horde of other NICU team members in tow, you're expecting to encounter one of those <1% scenarios. Imagine bursting through the Labor and Delivery unit's double doors and invariably finding no fewer than three members of the OB-GYN team waiting to point the way to where you're needed. In this circumstance, you're the cavalry and everyone is incredibly excited to see you.

When you and the rest of the NICU team get to room 5407, you're met at the door with a pair of gloves and a blue, limp, and silent baby lying on the warmer bed. Babies aren't supposed to be blue, or limp, or silent—they're supposed to be pink, thrashing, and screaming. I don't care how many newborns you've resuscitated, there's a moment that's uniquely jarring when you step to the head of a warmer bed surrounded by the friends and family of brand-new parents and begin resuscitating an infant whose entire body is the color of a week-old bruise.

I've always been grateful at times like these that much of the medicine we practice during a "code" situation is protocolized. It's rare for newborns not to respond to some part of the Neonatal Resuscitation Protocol (NRP), a step-by-step algorithm created and maintained by an expert group from the American Academy of Pediatrics. The NRP algorithm walks a code team and its leader sequentially through the interventions that evidence shows has the greatest likelihood of succeeding in saving an infant's life. While I learned the basics of NRP during my NICU rotations in residency, in fellowship the NRP pathway became deeply and permanently ingrained in the sulcations of my brain.

The NRP pathway begins just like I described for "STAT" page deliveries with warming, drying, bulb suction, and stimulation. While in old television shows the "stimulation" portion involved a doctor picking an infant up by the feet and whacking his tushy until he cried, that approach is generally frowned upon today. Instead, you would vigorously stroke the baby's back or flick his feet, though the vigor of such flicking markedly increases when the baby is blue.

Most babies will respond just to these steps within the first 30 seconds. For a baby who doesn't respond to your vigorous efforts to rub his back, flick his feet, and towel his head dry, you then place your fingers at the base of his umbilical cord (which feels like a very thick Twizzler) and feel for a pulse. If the baby's heart rate is below 100 beats per minute—which NRP instructors have classically taught is about the same rate as tapping out the beat to the classic Bee Gees song "Stayin' Alive"—you begin giving the baby rescue breaths. Staring at a blue newborn and knowing you are accountable for saving his life will send your own pulse well over 100 beats per minute, so you need to be mindful not to squeeze the base of an umbilical cord so hard that you feel your own pulse through your fingers instead of his.

Again, the vast majority of babies who don't respond to simulation will still respond to rescue breaths within the next 30-60 seconds, as the positive air pressure being blown into their lungs stimulates them to breathe, cry, and begin the normal transition to life outside of the womb. If, however, the baby doesn't respond, now is the time to contemplate intubation. As noted in Chapter 2, intubation involves placing a breathing tube through the baby's mouth and directly into his windpipe, allowing you to totally control his airway and avoid problems that come with pushing lots of air into the stomach (like vomit). The easiest intubations I've ever performed have been in situations like these, where the baby is totally limp and his life is entirely dependent on your placing the drinking-straw-sized tube perfectly through his tiny vocal cords. It's a high-stakes procedure but one that the vast majority of newborns who haven't yet turned around will respond to, bringing their heart rates up over 100 and sooner or later beginning to cry.

For those who still do not respond and whose heart rates fall to less than 60 beats per minute, the NRP algorithm directs you to now begin giving chest compressions. Of all the things I've simulated in medicine, performing newborn chest compressions comes the closest to feeling the same on a real baby as it does on a mannequin. While the same is not true for adult chest compressions, whoever makes newborn resuscitation simulation babies deserves a gold star.

Giving CPR to a newborn involves encircling his chest with your hands and squeezing his breastbone with your thumbs. Again, this is a somewhat jarring experience the first time you actually perform it because squeezing a baby just doesn't feel right under any circumstances. That said, knowing that CPR is in fact the only circumstance under which intentionally squeezing a baby won't get you arrested, you soldier on to the rhythm of the Bee Gees hoping the electric beeps of the heart monitor will soon pick up speed so you can stop.

At this point, if the baby hasn't responding to warming, drying, stimulation, positive pressure ventilation, intubation, and chest compressions, your odds of turning the corner begin to rapidly decrease. The next steps involve giving the stimulant medication epinephrine (which is the same thing as adrenaline) either directly into the breathing tube or into the baby's bloodstream through an emergency umbilical venous line. While an adult experiencing cardiac arrest needs an experienced doctor or nurse to find an adequately large vein in a hand, arm, neck, or groin to give code medications through, babies are conveniently born with umbilical cords. Umbilical cords come handily equipped with two arteries and one gigantic vein that can be used in an emergency resuscitation. A quick tie at the base of the cord to prevent spurting, a quick wipe with a chlorhexidine sponge to clean off the goo, a quick slice through the cord with a 15-blade scalpel (umbilical cords have no nerves so this isn't painful to the baby), and there you have it.

In cross-section, an umbilical cord sort of looks like a surprised-face emoji—the arteries are the two small eyes and the gaping, floppy-looking mouth at the bottom is the vein. You flush your line, take aim, and advance the catheter around 4-5 centimeters into the cord until you pull back on the attached syringe and get blood return. It's just that simple, except you're doing it to a baby who's still blue at the same time someone else is giving him CPR, a third person is holding and simultaneously securing the breathing tube, a fourth person is giving rescue breaths with either an AMBU bag or a T-piece resuscitator through that breathing tube, at least four other members of the code team are documenting, pulling medications, checking for a pulse, and watching the monitor for some sign of life, and an incredibly nervous set of parents, family members, and Labor and Delivery staff are watching your every move.

If epinephrine is going to work, it generally works pretty fast, so as soon as you've secured access you give a dose down the emergency umbilical venous line. After a few minutes with no change in the baby's heart rate, you give a second dose, and then a third. You try giving a bolus of intravenous normal saline because sometimes this works for infants who experience a sudden loss of blood during the delivery process. In this case it doesn't, so you're now 20 minutes in and still the baby is blue. By now your window to find a successful intervention is rapidly closing. You listen carefully to the baby's chest to see if he has a pneumothorax, you look inside his throat to make sure the breathing tube is exactly where it's supposed to be, you send STAT blood off to the lab to test for any abnormalities you could quickly correct, all the while giving more epinephrine, more intravenous fluid, more CPR, and more breaths.

In my entire career as a doctor, I've been in fewer than 10 delivery room codes that got this far without any response. While NRP doesn't explicitly tell you when to stop, it does say that "After ten minutes of continuous and adequate resuscitative efforts, discontinuation of resuscitation may be justified if there are no signs of life."[2] Ten minutes goes by very, very quickly when you are trying to save a newborn. I've had colleagues work a code on a term newborn for nearly an hour. A neonatal nurse practitioner I worked with said she once had a NICU fellow yell at her around the 30-minute mark to "Give a big-ass dose of epi!" She responded with "What do you mean a big-ass dose?" and he said "I don't care, just pull up a big-ass dose in a big-ass syringe and push it!" Having to declare a newborn dead is a special kind of hell that only those who've been there can appreciate, so such dramatic scenarios are rare but not unheard of only because trying anything at that point seems like a better option than calling the code.

Calling a code—or directing the team to stop resuscitation and declaring "time of death"—on a newborn baby must only be rivaled in agony by calling a code on a new mother. I remember responding to an "OB EMER" page one night in fellowship while on the phone coordinating a transport for an exceptionally sick infant from an outside hospital. I went running toward the Labor and Delivery operating rooms to find a senior neonatal nurse practitioner with a crying baby who looked completely healthy. I was still on the phone when the nurse practitioner waved me off, so without a second thought I went back into the unit to finalize the outside hospital transfer. That's when it hit me that this "OB EMER" page wasn't for us—it was for the mother.

During a caesarian section delivery, generally once a newborn has been warmed, dried, and cleaned up and after the pediatrics team has assigned the one- and five-minute APGAR scores, if everything looks good, the Labor and Delivery team assumes care for a newborn in the operating room. In this case, our NICU team stayed with the baby in the operating room while every member of the Labor and Delivery team went to the mattresses trying to save the mother. Hours went by, and ultimately our team brought the baby over to the well-baby nursery without her parents as the case went on. Additional surgeons joined the team, surrounding the new mother with experience from every surgical discipline on the small chance that someone had a unique skill or an idea that could make a difference. The team finally left the Labor and Delivery operating theatre late in the night, and took her to a different operating suite where even more advanced surgical techniques could be used. Nothing worked, and she died just hours after becoming a mother.

Later, during the very early morning hours, I joined the nurses who walked back to restock our newborn resuscitation area and noted that the Labor and Delivery operating room hadn't yet been cleaned. It actually hadn't even been touched since the massive team moved the new mother to the more advanced operating room on another floor of the hospital in a last desperate attempt to save her life. It's a sight that remains burned into my retinas to this day. The surgical table was still assembled, stabilizers still attached, and equipment strewn about the room as if hit by a hurricane. The pile of empty plastic bags on the ground from transfused blood products was taller than the table and stretched as wide as a twin mattress. Even the ventilator still pulsed, the rhythmic expansion and contraction of its accordion-like diaphragm unaware that its charge had long since departed both the operating room and this earth.

While I can't remember exactly when during fellowship it happened, that night must have been not long after my wife had given birth to our second child. Both she and our daughter Ellie had been thankfully perfectly healthy, and I very clearly remember thinking I couldn't conceive the pain of the man who had both become a father and lost his wife in the span of half a day. I could, however, deeply appreciate the pain of the doctors, surgeons, nurses, respiratory therapists, and every other member of the medical team who'd spent the best measures of their devotion over countless hours in a failed attempt to save the woman. New mothers, like newborns, are just not supposed to die.

I can count on one hand the number of newborn codes I've had to call in the delivery room. All of the infants were extremely premature, all born under incredibly unfortunate yet different circumstances, and none had a meaningful chance of surviving delivery (much less to discharge) even before they were born. That said, being premature doesn't make a baby any less human or any less loved, and each set of parents grieved in a way that only those who've experienced birth and death in such close proximity can truly appreciate.

The very first time I had to call a newborn code was in the middle of NICU fellowship. We had responded to an "OB EMER" page in the Labor and Delivery triage area, where a woman had just walked in and immediately given birth to a lifeless extremely premature infant. I was on call that night with one of the best nurse practitioners I will ever work with, and she had the tiny baby intubated within seconds. As the team began the resuscitation, I spoke with the OB-GYN resident and the mother to try to get any details I could about her history. I quickly learned that she was around 25 weeks pregnant and was visiting from another part of the state. Her regular OB-GYN had told her the baby "had some genetic problems" but she couldn't remember what they were other than that they were pretty serious.

A few minutes later into the code, the OB-GYN resident came back with more information, and it became clear that the infant was not only extremely premature but also had both a fatal genetic condition and an enormous congenital heart defect. What's more, after 20 minutes of CPR, the likelihood of any extremely premature infant surviving—much less one with the intractable challenges this particular baby faced—drops to near zero as the risk of a massive brain hemorrhage rises exponentially. I briefly conferred with the code team, then stepped to the mother's bed, explained to her the situation, and we both agreed it was time to stop resuscitation and transition to comfort care.

While the infant had never had a long-term life-sustaining heart rhythm, he did have a very, very slow heart rate and we had just given him several rounds of the heart-stimulating medication epinephrine. With the decision made to transition to comfort care, we stopped CPR, removed the breathing tube, swaddled him tightly, and brought all 500 grams of him over to his mother to hold. Since he still had a very slow heartbeat, we left them to bond and I returned every few minutes or so to listen again to his chest. It took almost an hour for his heart to stop completely. When it did, I removed the bell of my stethoscope from his tiny chest, looked gently up at his mother, and told her that he had died.

Over the next two hours, I learned that a lot had changed for me since my days as an emergency department technician when I first met death. Now, instead of being responsible for preparing the baby's body for the morgue (a process universally done by nurses in the Duke NICU and involving a shoebox-sized transport casket instead of a large metal slide), I had to try to draw blood from the infant's umbilical cord to confirm his suspected genetic condition. This was exceptionally harder than I expected but exceptionally important to get right, as the ramifications for his parents should they consider trying to get pregnant again could be critical. After we finally got the blood, the NICU nurses completed what I can only describe as a ritualistic process of taking handprints, footprints, and making other crucial memories for grieving parents to remember their newborn's life. I was standing by the fellow's station as these rituals were in progress when a team member from "Decedent Services" brought me a paper to sign. It was a death certificate. I'd seen other doctors sign them during residency, but there was always someone more senior than me involved in the handful of cases where a child died who took responsibility for signing it. This time, that most senior doctor wound up being me.

One of my favorite axioms comes from General Colin Powell, who says "when you're in charge, take charge." With this in mind I took the paper, sat at the fellow's desk in the main NICU workstation, and started to read it. I discovered that the top portion of a North Carolina death certificate is easy to complete, including basic demographic data like gender, first name, last name, date of birth, date of death, and time of death. The middle section included questions that were of limited utility in the NICU like "what was the decedent's occupation" and "did the decedent use tobacco." The final section, though, seemed rather important—it asked for the doctor to state the "immediate" cause of death, and then provided a handful of additional lines to enumerate other causes of death that sequentially led to the most immediate cause of death.

As there was no class in medical school or rotation in residency that taught "how to list causes of death," and since every human being in the history of the world has most immediately died of "cardiopulmonary failure" (meaning their heart and lungs both stopped), that's what I listed first. Figuring that was too broad to be the only cause of death, I then listed "presumed massive congenital heart defect" and "extreme prematurity" as additional diagnoses that led to cardiopulmonary failure, affixed my signature to the bottom, and handed it back. I've thought about that paper and its list of diagnoses for years, wondering if someday St. Peter will use it (and every other death certificate I've signed since) to stop me on the way to my own final judgment and assess my clinical acumen. They were all, of course, my best assessments at the time each baby died, but since most NICU deaths do not proceed to autopsy, they seemed really, really important to get right.

While deaths inside the delivery room are thankfully rare, I've been involved in many, many more deaths outside of the delivery room and inside the NICU itself. At the time I completed my NICU training, the "limit of viability" was around 23 weeks gestation and our NICU policy (consistent with most national and international practice at the time) was to offer limited resuscitation beginning for babies born at 23 weeks and 0 days. Even then, resuscitating a 23-and-0-week newborn wasn't without ethical challenges, as the best available data from the National Institutes of Health Neonatal Research Network suggested a best-case scenario of around 25% overall survival, and a much lower chance of survival without some kind of long-term debilitating medical problem.

The option to even try resuscitating a baby born this early is the handiwork of just the most recent generation of doctors and scientists. In 1963, First Lady Jackie Kennedy gave birth to a premature son named Patrick. He died on his second day of life from something called "hyaline membrane disease," a condition that at the time had no known cause and no known cure. He was only five weeks early, weighed almost 5 pounds, had access to the best possible medical care with no barriers to cost or access, and still died.

Five decades and countless advances in care for preemies later funded by both public institutions (e.g., the National Institute of Child Health and Human Development) and private entities (e.g., March of Dimes), Patrick Bouvier Kennedy would today have a nearly 100% chance of surviving. Not only would he likely survive, but he would tower over the other infants in the NICU like a giant among men. As a neonatologist in the 2010s, I've cared for infants born three times earlier and six times smaller than Patrick Kennedy and they've made it home alive and well. The youngest infant I've helped care for in the NICU was born four months early. The smallest weighed about the same as a can of soda. Both are now boisterous preschoolers.

Each of these advances in care for preemies—e.g., the invention of umbilical lines, the discovery and isolation of a substance called surfactant that can help open very premature lungs, and the evolution of ventilators able to support extraordinarily small lungs without repeatedly popping them—pushed the "limit of viability" earlier and earlier into a mother's pregnancy. Yet no matter how far we push, there remains a line beyond which technology has yet to reach. Furthermore, while today's science and technology mean we can give 24-, 23-, and even arguably 22-weekers a meaningful chance of survival, there are many preemies who still do not survive their NICU stays.

Given those odds, over the last 10 years I have been involved in nearly a hundred discussions with families about "withdrawing" or "transitioning to comfort care." These conversations are rarely a surprise, as NICU teams work hard to stay in very close contact with families over the course of an extremely premature or extremely sick newborn's stay. Through both daily family-centered rounds—where parents join the whole rounding team's discussion about each day's plan of care—to more formal "family meetings," NICU parents and NICU teams develop a shared understanding of how to define the inflection point. While its exact location is different for each set of parents, all families share the common existence of some signal that says "we are no longer doing things for the baby and instead only doing things to the baby."

The most memorable of these conversations for me involved a family I'd grown to know well over a few days on-service near the end of my fellowship. The baby's name was Sam* and he had been born around 16 weeks early. Sam was critically ill from the start, born in septic shock with a severe bacterial infection raging through his tiny body that we were unlikely to be able to get under control. That said, his parents and our team agreed we would try as hard as we could anyway. We gave him nearly every therapy the NICU had to offer, including high-frequency ventilation, pure oxygen mixed with nitric oxide, massive doses of intravenous antibiotics and medications to support his blood pressure, and multiple blood transfusions. He was ridiculously sick but barely holding on when on his third day of life his body's posture significantly changed. Instead of lying curled up in the fetal position, he extended his arms outward at an awkwardly straight angle. His entire body then became rigid and his gaze went from fighting to blank. Concerned for the worst, we ordered a STAT ultrasound of his brain. The imaging study confirmed the worst-case scenario: a large, active intraventricular bleed inside his brain that would be impossible for him to survive.

By that point, Sam's parents and I had ridden the ups and downs of his rollercoaster together for three days, knowing we'd sooner or later likely come to this most gut-wrenching curve in the track. They asked how long he could still survive on the mammoth doses of medications and the other specialized treatments, and I answered likely hours at best. They asked me how long he would survive without them, and I answered minutes, maybe even seconds. That's all it took. We kept him on the menagerie of NICU technology surrounding his tiny isolette until they could rally their whole family to the hospital. Once prepared, Sam's nurse disconnected all but the one medication line he had for pain and sedation, and the respiratory therapist helped me switch him off the high-frequency ventilator. I picked his tiny body up and cradled him in my arm, using a hand-powered AMBU bag to breathe for him during the 40-foot walk from his isolette to the room we'd prepared for his family. He stayed alive through the trip, but only barely.

When we got to the packed room, I very gently passed Sam over to his mother, who nuzzled her baby's face and touched him bare-handed for the first time. He met his siblings, his grandparents, his aunts, and his uncles. His father held him as he completed the trip around the family room, while I kept periodically giving him hand-powered breaths with the AMBU bag through his breathing tube. Once they were ready to let go, we returned Sam to his mother's arms, disconnected the AMBU bag, and using a special adhesive-remover swab, I very carefully removed the tape that secured his breathing tube. I then pulled out the tube, his face now totally free of medical equipment for the first time since he emerged from his mother's womb. He died seconds later. In the words of Ronald Reagan, he "slipped the surly bonds of earth to touch the face of God" while wrapped within the love of his mother's deep embrace.

Of all the families I've helped walk through these kinds of final hours, I remember this one most clearly because it was the most personally involved I've ever been in the final minutes of a person's life. Sam's parents and I made the decision together that it was time to transition to comfort care. I carried Sam out of the NICU and into the family room personally, I manually gave him his last breath, and I removed the breathing tube that only barely sustained his life. I went home that day and wrapped my arms around each of my own children. I am convinced that on that day and every day thereafter, I've hugged all three of them a little harder than I did before I met Sam and his incredible family.

With three years of fellowship having regularly brought me into very close proximity with both birth and death, my wife's third pregnancy in my final year of training involved nine months of near-constant fret. Melody tells me I'm lucky she didn't know how hard it would be for her to be pregnant with a neonatologist's baby because it may have been a deal-breaker. By the time she made it to 20 weeks gestation in the fall of 2013 and the ultrasound looked good, we basically stopped talking about my work for the next 20 weeks out of both superstition and to preserve our sanity.

My youngest child John wound up being born healthy and at term on a Sunday. My wife's water broke at home around 3 a.m. that morning, and our neighbors drove down to stay with our older two until my in-laws could come to take over. We hightailed it to Durham Regional, the hospital whose Special Care Nursery I enjoyed working in so much and where her OB-GYN group had privileges to deliver babies. We were registered in the Labor and Delivery triage around 4 a.m. and made it to a room around 5. By this point I'd seen hundreds if not thousands of heart rate and uterine contraction tracings, and while I'm not an OB-GYN, I could tell that things looked good and seemed to be moving along fairly fast. With our first child my wife labored for nearly 12 hours and pushed for more than two. With our second she had labored for only a few hours and pushed for a matter of minutes. Our third would be a boy, and he seemed to be in much more of a rush than either of his sisters.

The OB-GYN came in, an attending and a partner from another group in town who traded call with my wife's practice. I knew him well from joining the Special Care Nursery's delivery team on overnight moonlighting shifts for many of his patients. He checked everything, said Melody and the baby both looked great, and since she was only 5-6 centimeters dilated (a cervix needs to be around 10 centimeters dilated to be ready for delivery), he was going to take a shower while the anesthesia team placed the epidural.

He left the room and moments later an anesthesiologist walked in and began setting up her tray. As she began asking her standard pre-procedural questions, my wife said she "felt some pressure." The anesthesiologist paused her rote questioning and stepped out to get the Labor and Delivery nurse, who promptly checked my wife again and found my son's head already crowning. To this day I have no idea how, but that anesthesiologist melted away as quickly and quietly as any human being has ever moved on the face of the earth, because in the seconds after my eyes went from the nurse to my wife, she had vanished.

With no time for an epidural and no stopping my son from entering the world on his own time, the nurse stepped to the foot of the bed and prepared to catch him. As the only doctor in the room, I felt momentarily paralyzed wondering whether I needed to step up with the nurse and help deliver my own son. Remembering the last slippery newborn I had to catch as a medical student, I figured that would be unwise, and with the skilled Labor and Delivery nurse temporizing matters, I ran to the hallway and yelled "we need a doctor in here now!"

One of the second-year OB-GYN residents I knew from working with him at Duke tore out of the work-station and down the hall, busting through the door to our Labor and Delivery suite with a look of purpose. He quickly glanced around and, presuming my son was stuck mid-delivery with a condition called a shoulder dystocia, asked the nurse, "Have you tried the McRoberts maneuver yet?" She looked him square in the eye, my son's head now fully delivered and said, "No, you idiot, he's not stuck. He's just ready to come now!"

The resident then immediately understood and, bare-handed, took his seat in the rolling stool at the foot of my wife's bed. With a single push, the rest of my son came flying out of the womb—the resident deftly caught him, flipped the boy up on his mother's chest,

stepped to the sink, and calmly washed his hands. Total shock doesn't begin to describe the look on Melody's face when her glance moved from the glistening,
screaming newborn on her chest up to me, her eyes saying, "What the f-ck just happened?"

I've been present for hundreds of deliveries before
and after that day, yet my son remains the only newborn I've ever seen caught barehanded by an OB-GYN
resident. An auspicious birth to say the least, and one
that I am certain neither the Durham Regional Labor
and Delivery nurse nor the resident (who by now must
be an attending OB-GYN somewhere in America) will
forget anytime soon.

— 5 —

The Bottom of the Well

"Happiness can be found, even in the darkest of times, if one only remembers to turn on the light."

–Dumbledore: *Harry Potter and the Prisoner of Azkaban*

It started with a bitter taste in my mouth. I was nearing hour 27 of an in-house call as a pediatrics resident, and had just broken away from morning rounds to return a "911" page from the radiology department. I've returned a lot of 911 pages and, while the person on the other end of the line is always rather animated, on this particular morning the phone was answered by an exceptionally concerned attending pediatric radiologist. "I'm looking at this kid's film from overnight," she began, "and it looks there's a huge mass hiding in the middle of one of the images. I don't see where the radiology team discussed this with you guys at all on the night shift... you know that it's there, right?"

I knew the patient she was calling about and had, in fact, looked at the same film myself very late the previous night. I remember something about the radiograph hadn't looked completely normal to me and I asked a more senior resident to look at it too. Neither of us could put our finger on exactly what bothered us, and we'd gone to bed awaiting the pediatric radiologist's final report in the morning. What we didn't expect was that "something funny" wound up being a tumor hiding in plain sight.

I remember noticing the bitter taste immediately upon hearing the words "huge mass," followed by feeling like my heart would pound out of my chest and a combination of dizziness and confusion reserved only for those who've visited hour 27 of continuous wakefulness. I hadn't pushed to follow up on the gut twitch I had looking at the film the night before, and in doing so had made a mistake. On a normal day a finding like this wouldn't be an overnight urgency. However, the ramifications in this case were potentially catastrophic because that particular patient on that particular day was by then already undergoing a procedure whose risk could be dramatically increased by the presence of such a hidden tumor.

It took barely a minute for the epinephrine squeezed from my adrenal glands to complete its course through my bloodstream, first igniting the bitter taste, the dizziness, and the hammering heartbeat. Upon finally reaching my brain, the epinephrine reignited my sleepy synapses and I snapped from dizzy confusion into hyper alert attention. Recognizing our patient's potential peril, I sprinted off the pediatrics unit, took the stairs three at a time up several floors, and launched into the procedure room's unsterile ante chamber to alert the team. Incredibly, the patient was completely fine. But in that moment, bleary-eyed and holding my old-school flip phone with a now distressed and very confused radiologist still squawking into the other end, the weight of that mistake felt crushing.

Mistakes are not only part of medicine—they are, in fact, inevitable. Doctors, nurses, physical therapists, and all other healthcare providers are human. While we may be very specially trained humans, just like the billions of other humans on this planet, we are all fallible.

During medical school, I didn't learn much about making mistakes, what to do about them, or what we as individual doctors could do to prevent them beyond "just be a better doctor." I also didn't appreciate the sheer magnitude of harm seemingly minor mistakes could cause until a nondescript lunch lecture I attended during residency in the weeks following the "911" page. The lecture was on a Tuesday, the most popular day of the week for lunch lectures among Duke's pediatric residents because the free food came from a Durham staple called Cosmic Cantina. Known best for staying open until 4a.m. for all the undergrads "celebrating" Duke basketball wins into the wee hours of the morning, Cosmic Cantina also had decent burritos and our spectacular residency coordinator always made sure there was one for me without cheese.

On that particular Tuesday, I remember filing with the other residents into the cramped Department of Pediatrics' classroom with burrito in hand, thankful no one had accidentally pilfered its queso-less goodness. I settled into a chair while a PowerPoint slide titled "Adverse Events" blazed across the projector screen. At the time I couldn't define an "adverse event" to save my life, but I'd already busted into the burrito's foil wrapper and started chomping away by the time I'd read the slide, so I figured I might as well stick around to find out what it meant.

On a brief side note, I do not ever recommend trying to eat with a doctor. In medical school I learned to eat faster than the interns, and interns have to eat fast enough to beat their pagers' relentless beckoning. On my surgery rotation, my best performance involved pounding four chicken fingers, a plate of fries, and a 20-ounce Pepsi from Café Duke in 178 seconds. So when I say "started chomping away," I really mean it. It's a habit that 10 years in practice and living with three kids of my own under the age of 10 has done nothing to deter.

Back to residency, within minutes the classroom reached its stifling capacity and one of our chief residents stepped to the podium. She apologized that the professor planning to lecture that day on Henoch-Schonlein Purpura—a condition that even today I still cannot understand or explain—had to back out at the last minute. There had been some kind of "emergency" in his basic science laboratory and he couldn't leave, which left me wondering if a dangerous strain of mutant virus or a dangerous army of mutant mice (or God forbid both) was now roaming the halls of the research building en route to the hospital. Instead, she announced, she'd be giving the lunch lecture and was going to talk to us about quality improvement and patient safety.

She began the lecture by explaining the basic tenets of healthcare's patient safety movement, starting with the Institute of Medicine's landmark reports *To Err is Human* in 1999 and *Crossing the Quality Chasm* in 2001. She introduced phrases like "preventable harm" and "continuous improvement," words that then sounded totally out of place to me in clinical practice but over the next decade I would come to know and use intimately. At the time, though, I was only halfway paying attention to her defining "adverse event" and halfway thinking about the cardiology service I was covering, which included a few kids with heart rhythm problems, one who'd been through no less than four open heart surgeries, and even a child who'd received a heart transplant.

I was particularly focused on the heart transplant patient. He had received the transplant some years prior, and needed to be admitted from time to time for a "tune up" to his various medication regimens and to undergo a variety of tests to ensure his transplanted heart was still functioning well. He was almost ready for discharge, so I was running through my mental list of things I'd need to do to get him home before the weekend when the chief resident started giving examples of real patient safety events reported in the medical literature. One nearly made me choke on my already largely devoured Cosmic burrito.

She told the story of a patient at a well-respected hospital who was receiving sodium supplements. Sodium chloride is the same thing as table salt, and is a fairly common supplement in both pediatric and adult medicine. For example, some medications used to treat heart failure cause a patient's kidneys to waste extra sodium. Since the kidneys are the primary organ our bodies use to balance the salt and water content in our blood, wasting too much sodium in the urine can drive a patient's bloodstream sodium levels dangerously low. To prevent this from happening, rather than asking patients to douse their lunches with salt, we give them carefully measured sodium supplements to balance the amount that the kidneys waste. In this case, however, an error involving simple table salt led to catastrophic consequences.

Sodium supplements generally come in a clear syringe that contains a clear, colorless, odorless liquid composed of dissolved sodium chloride and water. As best as the team could ultimately figure out after the event, what instead reached this particular patient was a clear syringe labeled "sodium" but filled with a different colorless, odorless, and impossible-to-distinguish solution composed of potassium. Large doses of potassium rapidly lead to dangerous changes in the heart's electrical rhythm and can be challenging, if not impossible, to reverse. This patient apparently received the inadvertent dose of potassium, immediately experienced a fatal heart rhythm, went into cardiac arrest, and died.

Even worse, the chief resident noted that this sodium/potassium substitution wasn't a one-time, one-hospital event—over a five-year period in the late 1990s, the Federal Drug Administration's Adverse Event Reporting System[3] reported 469 fatal medication errors. While most of those fatal errors involved inadvertent drug overdoses, 73 deaths involved patients receiving the wrong drug and eight of those specifically involved potassium, which caregivers across multiple hospitals in multiple states had accidentally given to patients instead of everything from sodium to blood thinners to heart failure medications. The final kicker was that the Food and Drug Administration's database was not only a decade old, but it only included voluntarily reported errors. This meant that the true burden of fatal medication errors was likely much, much higher than the "one every four days" that the authors had calculated.

To say I was stunned would be a colossal understatement. I was literally caring for a human being who had another human being's heart beating in his chest, the product of some of the most complex surgery and the

---

3   https://www.ncbi.nlm.nih.gov/pubmed/11596700

most complex medicine ever practiced in the history of humanity. And yet in the same era, at the same time, that same advanced medicine hadn't yet found a way to prevent simple human error from killing hundreds of patients by mistaking something as simple as potash for table salt. If we could transplant a heart, this seemed to me like something we as a profession needed to and could fix.

Given the millions of medications patients receive every day at hospitals around the nation, it shouldn't be surprising that medication errors are some of the most common mistakes in healthcare. In 10 years as a doctor, I've now written thousands of medication orders and I've made my share of prescribing errors. The vast majority of these errors were caught by the hospital or clinic's electronic medical record's computerized ordering system before I even submitted the prescription. A common example would be substituting milligrams per kilogram (mg/kg) for micrograms per kilogram (mcg/kg). That one "c" yields a 1,000-fold difference in dose, or roughly the same as replacing a banded mongoose with a giraffe. Another example would be accidentally replacing one look-alike/sound-alike drug with another, like dexamethasone (a steroid) with dextromethorphan (a cough suppressant). Well-tuned computerized order entry systems offer something called clinical decision support, which is an automated way to catch errors like this and alert either the prescriber or the pharmacist to correct the order before it even gets prepared, much less dispensed or actually delivered to a patient.

I have, of course, also made errors in prescribing medications that the electronic medical record hasn't caught. Of those, the vast majority were caught by another member of the healthcare team before they reached a patient. I have more than once discussed starting a premature infant on a diuretic medication, a drug that helps remove extra fluid from a baby's lungs by increasing the amount of urine made by the kidneys, only to inadvertently enter the order to start the next morning. Called by the nurse who usually says something like "Doctor Chris, didn't you mean to start the Lasix today?" I've gone back to correct the order, thanked the nurse, and again been humbled that practicing medicine is now and always has been truly a team sport.

The most egregious error I've ever made when ordering a medication was caught by a pharmacist and thankfully never reached a patient. It happened one night when I was in the middle of residency. I was cross-covering the entire pediatrics unit, and one of the day-shift residents had asked me to order precautionary emergency medications for a cancer patient to have ready for his chemotherapy for the following day. Certain chemotherapy regimens can cause an immediate and life-threatening allergic reaction. While such reactions are exceptionally rare, they are also exceptionally dangerous, so whenever patients receive these drug combinations, we also order a series of preemptive emergency medication orders that most often go unused. These "held" orders sit dormant in the electronic order system, tagged to the patient with pre-calculated weight-based doses ready to go in case a nurse delivering the chemo needs to emergently activate them in the setting of such a reaction.

You might ask, "Why not wait the few minutes it would take for a doctor to come to the bedside?" Seconds matter during an anaphylactic reaction, and waiting just a few minutes to begin treatment could be fatal. That said, such chemotherapy regimens are so common that entering emergency medication orders for a pediatrics resident cross-covering a cancer service becomes routine. The process becomes so routine, in fact, that I could literally enter them in my sleep—which that night is close to what happened. We'd had an incredibly busy call with lots of admissions, including bringing several children coming up from the emergency department and transferring in others directly to the floor from other hospitals. It was after 2 a.m. by the time I finally made my way to the call room for a short nap before beginning morning pre-rounds.

As my head hit the pillow, with the promise of sleep now merely seconds away, I remembered I still had to enter the cancer patient's emergency medications for the next day. I pulled a rolling chair up next to the call room's desktop computer, logged in, opened the patient's chart, and entered the orders—intravenous diphenhydramine, prednisone, and epinephrine. It took me maybe 45 seconds to write, double-check, and sign the orders, and then I went to bed. Call room beds feel like lying on plywood and smell like a college dorm, but that didn't matter. Residency had taught me to sleep anywhere on anything at any time. I was out cold before the computer finished its shutdown sequence.

Around 20 minutes into my heavily laden sleep, I was paged by a pharmacist. In most leading teaching hospitals, unless a medication is ordered, drawn, and given at the bedside under urgent circumstances, medication orders are reviewed and approved by a pharmacist before being prepared, double-checked again, and dispensed to the bedside for a nurse to administer. In this case, a pediatric pharmacist happened to be working the night shift who was familiar with pediatric precautionary emergency medication orders. She also knew that the correct epinephrine dose for emergency medications was 0.01mg/kg. I had entered 0.1mg/kg, a 10-fold overdose that would have been potentially disastrous had it been put to use.

When I called back the number on my pager, the pharmacist had every right to have answered the phone and screamed, "DeRienzo, ARE YOU CRAZY?!? If I hadn't caught your EPIC screw-up and God forbid the patient got this drug, you could have killed him!" But she didn't. We knew each other well, and she knew that I was about as conscientious a resident as has walked the face of the earth. On most days I obsessively checked and rechecked my orders and circled back behind the more junior residents under my watch to make sure their orders too were accurate. She also knew that I was a human. And that night, no matter how obsessively compulsive she could generally count on me to be on a normal day, I was fallible and had made a very dangerous mistake.

Instead of reaming me out, she said, "Chris, sorry to wake you up, but I was looking at your emergency medication orders and I think you meant to order the epinephrine at 0.01mg/kg instead of 0.1mg/kg." My heart rate rapidly accelerated from sleep to overdrive, as if I'd just been given the wallop of epinephrine I'd accidentally ordered for the patient, as the latent impact of my error sank in. I said, "Oh my God you're right, thank you so much." She said she would fix the order using the pharmacy's order entry system and sent me back to bed. I thanked her again for catching my mistake, and once more revelled in the team-based nature of practicing medicine.

It's simply an unavoidable fact that *all* people— even the most Type A, neurotic, or well-trained and well-meaning people—make mistakes. Every doctor has a personal responsibility to train as hard as she can, stay as sharp and current as she can, and focus her energy and attention on each individual patient as diligently as she can. Yet there exists no amount of training, focus, energy, or diligence to prevent 100% of human errors.

For centuries, physicians refused to publicly acknowledge our fallibility. Instead, we taught medical students and residents that making a mistake was tantamount to a profound personal failure. We actively cultivated an aura of error-free perfection and hid our mistakes from the rest of the world. Behind closed doors, doctors in training who made mistakes were systematically chastised inside the chambers of morbidity and mortality (M&M) conferences. Such M&M sessions historically involved facing a firing squad of senior physicians intended to so humiliate and excoriate the trainee as to prevent any mistake from ever happening again.

This deep-seated cultural resistance to admitting our own failures has left medicine way behind in adapting to the concept of systematic safety that industries like nuclear power, commercial air travel, and manufacturing have embraced for decades. Despite this façade, our entire profession has, in fact, committed colossal and very public mistakes, some of which have lasted for centuries. Remember blood-letting? Oops. How about leeches? Unless you have a severely necrotic wound—for which there is now unbelievably a real treatment that involves sterile, biomedically prepared leeches—we wasted about a thousand years using the little parasitic bloodsuckers to treat everything from sciatica to "humoral imbalances." For a more modern example, consider the hundreds of drugs from the 20th century that we thought we were using to treat disease but were actually causing harm. Just Google "thalidomide," "cis-apride," or "diethylstilbestrol," and you'll get a sense of what I mean.

All that said, the most incredible mistakes we've made as a medical profession involve failing to adopt the rare new practice that clearly defines a stairstep toward a better standard of care. I'm not talking about the hundreds of novel therapies published in the medical literature every day, though I'll touch on that later in the book. Instead, I mean truly world-changing advances that happen perhaps once or twice a century. Here's just one example.

Imagine it's 1846 and we're in Vienna. You've just given birth and are waiting in your "child bed" to see the physician team, totally blind to the fact that you have a three times greater chance of dying (about 1 in 10) than the woman next to you being cared for by a midwife (about 1 in 33). Now fast-forward two years. You survived your first pregnancy and have returned to the same maternity ward to deliver your second baby. It's now 1848, and after a stunning discovery by an OB-GYN named Dr. Ignaz Semmelweis, your chances of dying have dramatically dropped. Now, whether you are cared for by a physician or a midwife, instead of a 1 in 10 or a 1 in 33 chance of dying, you now have a 99% chance of survival.

Why? Because Dr. Semmelweis discovered that to prevent the spread of "puerperal fever"—now known to be caused by an overwhelming bacterial infection—physicians just had to wash their hands. Said Dr. Semmelweis in his 1861 paper:

"Even so, one cannot impute guilt… any more than to me or to all the others who undertook examinations with contaminated hands. *None of us knew that we were causing the numerous deaths."*

With such a dramatic change in outcomes after such a small change in practice, it would be reasonable to expect that Dr. Semmelweis was celebrated the world over, unifying medicine around hand hygiene as fast as information could travel in the mid-1800s. Reasonable, but wrong. Instead, Dr. Semmelweis was fired from his job and exiled from the Austrian medical community. He died four years later, having been committed to an asylum while women around the world continued dying at an unconscionable rate from a now clearly preventable condition.

Medicine has come a long way in the last 150 years. If you're giving birth in the U.S. today, you have a 99.98% chance of survival. Childhood leukemia—a once uniformly fatal condition—is survivable in over 80% of cases, and NICUs can save infants born more than four months early who weigh under a pound at birth. Yet in spite of such incredible advances in care, the "Semmelweis reflex"—an out-of-hand rejection of new information no matter how potentially transformative or ironclad its evidence—remains prevalent. Furthermore, despite 150 years of knowing better, we still can't reach 100% adherence to even the most 100% proven practices like washing our hands. As a result, the *Journal of Patient Safety's* most recently published estimate puts the number of deaths in healthcare caused by preventable harm at around 400,000 per year. Do the math—in just the time it's taken you to read this chapter, well-meaning and well-trained clinicians somewhere in America have inadvertently killed at least five people.

While today we remain far from perfect, at least we

have finally come to acknowledge as a community of physicians that we are not superhuman and will never be perfect. Whether we make a mistake once in every 10,000 actions, once in 100,000, or once in 1,000,000, sooner or later, every doctor makes a mistake. Instead of chastising those who make mistakes and hiding them from sight for fear of legal and professional consequences, it turns out the best way to meaningfully improve patient safety is to build systems that keep those inevitable errors from reaching patients and causing harm.

In the "Just Culture" model used by the world's safest and highest-performing hospitals and clinics, human error is understood to be a part of life and part of practice. Except in the rare circumstance where a clinician commits an error while under the influence of alcohol or drugs, intentionally injures someone, or purposefully skirts a well-defined and safe process, the Just Culture model instructs leaders to support the person who makes a mistake and fix the process that allows it to reach a patient. While all doctors remain responsible for their own actions and must work continually to refine their craft, the vast majority of errors that reach patients and cause harm involve countless system failures that fixing the person involved will never prevent. The Just Culture model teaches that if a similarly trained clinician could reasonably be placed in circumstances similar to those of a clinician involved in an adverse event and make the same mistake, then by definition the process—not the person—needs improvement.

This Just Culture concept resonated with me in a deeply personal way the day I first heard about it during the chief resident's lecture on Cosmic burrito day. I recalled the day that my red-light ambulance hands waved over the concrete stoop of my childhood home in New

York, trying to prevent my sister's inevitable death from eating berries off our backyard bush. I'd apparently been a patient safety advocate since preschool; I just didn't know it until residency.

Ten years later, I now get to spend much of my time as a physician leader working with teams across hospitals and clinics to prevent these kinds of errors. I've worked with teams involved in terribly tragic outcomes, and invariably the people involved all feel the same deep sense of failure that I felt that day in residency when I received the 911 radiology page. For all good clinicians—and I firmly believe that 99.9% of doctors, nurses, therapists, and so on are good people who come to clinical practice for good reasons—each mistake grates at your soul and takes an increasingly bigger bite out of your resiliency.

In his incredible book on life and death *When Breath Becomes Air*, the late Dr. Paul Kalanithi captured how this relentless grating erodes away at a clinician's personal sense of wellbeing:

"The cost of my dedication to succeed was high, and the ineluctable failures brought me nearly unbearable guilt. Those burdens are what make medicine holy and wholly impossible: *in taking up another's cross, one must sometimes get crushed by the weight.*"

For me, within weeks of that 911 page mistake as a resident—and despite the fact that the patient wasn't actually harmed—I was without question crushed by the weight. Unlike the immediacy of the epinephrine rush on the day I received that 911 page, the uneasiness that followed metastasized much more slowly yet became much more necrotic. I didn't realize it at the time, but I was experiencing all the symptoms that today we recognize as clinician burnout.

I was woefully sleep-deprived yet couldn't sleep, struggling just to survive each day in the hospital until I could sign out to the next resident. I was also shorter with people at work, and ultimately shorter at home as well. I began to strongly consider quitting medicine entirely, despite having invested decades into getting through college, medical school, and now residency. I went so far as to touch base with friends from years earlier who had gone into management consulting and started lining up options for an interview. The beginnings of such a profound personal and professional spiral left me feeling totally inept as a doctor, a husband, and generally speaking as a human being.

My experience during those months is not unique. Burnout in healthcare has by any definition reached epidemic proportions. According to the CDC's *Principles of Epidemiology*, an epidemic refers to "An increase, often sudden, in the number of cases above what is normally expected in [a] population." Few would argue that the explosion of evidence around burnout in healthcare falls short of "a sudden increase." In truth, one could actually quite reasonably argue whether recent data are, in fact, an increase "above what is normally expected" or whether burnout has been endemic but unmeasured in healthcare forever. It's hard to fathom why in a field that, by its nature demands a deep and constantly contested emotional well, it took this long for burnout in healthcare to hit the national consciousness.

Things obviously didn't start for me this way. Like all caregivers, I was "called to serve" a greater good in healthcare and began my career as a bright-eyed medical student keen on making the world a healthier place.

The bright glow of such a calling shines like an old coastal lighthouse, a beacon in the dark summoning clinicians home whenever they need to remember why they've chosen to serve in whatever area of healthcare they serve. Yet like a lighthouse, the shine of this calling can become obscured by layers of the grime of reality. Suffocating medical student debt often coats the bulb in its first dark film, which then gets thicker in the midst of working 80 hours a week in a state of perpetual sleep deprivation under a system of teaching young doctors that remains largely unchanged since the Taft administration.

Life's joys—family, friends, spiritual wholeness, and fulfillment in one's professional and personal goals to name a few—periodically help cleanse the grime, allowing one's purpose in medicine to again shine through and propelling a clinician back off the shore and again into the ocean's rough waters. It should be no surprise, however, that there comes a time in any clinician's career when the layers of grime are packed so thick that it wouldn't take much more to fully block the light from view. For me, the 911 page mistake I made in residency was such a tipping point. The ensuing darkness sent me into a tailspin that made me question to the core why I had worked so hard to become a doctor.

Unfortunately, the Just Culture approach to preventing human errors from reaching patients hadn't yet fully matured when I made my 911 page mistake as a resident. There was no system in place to bring me into the folds of a process-driven root cause analysis response team. No one reminded me that at least five other doctors had the opportunity to look at the same film I had seen and stop the line, and we kicked off no process improvement effort to enhance the pre-procedural evaluation or critical radiographic abnormality reporting pathways. Instead, I was alone, spiraling in circles around my own guilt just as legions of other physicians have done since Hippocrates. I spiraled until the Cosmic burrito lecture offered me an opportunity to see the world and my own mistake through a different lens. Whether she knows it or not, the chief resident's choice to focus that day's lecture on patient safety and preventing adverse events probably saved my career from taking a very, very different path. Having now worked with hundreds of clinicians who've made mistakes, I can say with certainty that we've learned a lot in the last decade about supporting clinicians through these kinds of tailspins. We also now know how to help build up clinicians' resiliency to burnout before they ever reach the precipice, and we know how to work as a team to understand why mistakes reach patients, root out underlying systemic failures, and find ways to fix them. We have acknowledged that mistakes put not only patients at risk of harm but clinicians at risk of reaching their own personal breaking points, and we've built even stronger systems to surround them with professional, collegial, and sometimes even formal psychological support.

I will never forget leading one root cause analysis team that involved multiple clinicians and a medication error. We spent hours together, and by the end of the root cause analysis process, we had identified a number of system failures that could have contributed to the medication error reaching the patient. The team was proud of our work, feeling confident that our actions would make the process safer for the next patient. On the final day, we began to wrap up and people started filing out of the conference room when I noticed one clinician crying uncontrollably.

Given the seriousness of the events teams discuss during a root cause analysis process—sometimes involving patients who experience serious preventable harm or even death—I've seen a lot of tears. Most often, though, team members working through root cause analysis cry during the beginning of the session as we talk through an event's chronology and each person adds their part of the story. I had never seen someone cry at the end, once the stories were told, the process errors identified, and interventions put in place to prevent them from happening again.

Feeling a bit startled, I walked up to the clinician to see if she was OK. She looked me in the eyes and said she'd come to the first meeting a few weeks prior fully expecting the entire team to call out her personal failure as the reason the patient experienced the error. She hadn't slept the night before and was terrified, but felt like she had to stand to account for her mistake and had fully prepared herself for the berating she anticipated would come. She felt deeply personally responsible, and entered the room thinking "if only I had been a better clinician and done this one thing differently, none of the rest would have happened."

Working through a root cause analysis doesn't make that statement false. There are often many people and many processes involved in an event where we wish "this one thing would have happened differently." And therein lies the magic. Having now reached the end, with no berating in sight, she still felt guilty but the difference was she no longer felt alone. We were all a team—clinicians and leaders alike—and we shared responsibility at every step of the way for the event that ultimately reached the patient.

This "Swiss Cheese" model of error was most famously described by the author James Reason in his groundbreaking book *Human Error*. Reason noted that every slice of Swiss cheese has a slightly different assortment of holes. If you randomly line up 10 slices of cheese all in a row, every so often you'll be able to find a set of holes that happen to align across them all. In medicine, when those metaphorical holes line up just right, an error can fall through them all and reach a patient. In the case of this particular error, the clinician now understood that she was only one slice of cheese. She'd started the day teetering on the verge of the same kind of collapse I'd begun to experience in residency. Thanks to James Reason, Just Culture, and the supportive senior leadership team needed for a health system to truly implement it, she ended it feeling whole again, able to once more see the light of her professional purpose.

One of my two favorite quotes comes from Sister Catherine McAuley. Sister McAuley founded the Sisters of Mercy nearly 200 years ago in Ireland to serve, shelter, and educate the poorest members of Irish society. Since then, her movement has expanded worldwide, covering many charitable works and at least two large Mercy health systems in the United States. In a letter she penned to Sister Mary de Sales in February 1841, she wrote: "The simplest and most practical lesson I know… is to resolve to be good today, but better tomorrow."

No two words, in my opinion, better capture the central objective in the practice of medicine than "getting better." Catherine McAuley's words remind us that— even as doctors—we are only human and therefore incapable of perfection. However, they also remind us that because we can never reach perfection, we will also never run out of opportunities to learn, grow, and improve. For some, that reality may seem depressing, but for me, it's incredibly inspiring and is, in fact, the reason Just Culture and root cause analysis are such useful tools in finding, fixing, and systematically addressing errors.

The best example I know of living these words comes from a great mentor of mine, Dr. Ronald Paulus. He once told me that on his childhood walks to school he sought each day to decrease the total number of steps he took by at least one. He spent months continuously redesigning his route and taking longer steps, ultimately diverting by year's end through a playground because he decided that traversing the monkey bars didn't count as "steps." I knew then that in Ron I'd found a kindred spirit, having similarly spent hours in my own childhood trying to find the most efficient way to carry my mass of Transformers toys from room to room. At the time, my mother always cautioned me not to "take the lazy man's load." Now I know that I wasn't being lazy –I've just been bent on driving continuous improvement since preschool.

In the NICU, this need to always get better at how we care for babies runs deep. Unlike the adult patients in a primary care clinic, our babies come into the world with no past medical histories, no responsibility for any of their health outcomes, and an enormous universe of potential harms that can befall them while hospitalized. Couple this with the fact that newborns, especially preemies, are the most vulnerable people on earth, and our NICU team is effectively genetically conditioned to protect and defend our babies.

In the late 1980s, one of the ways NICUs realized they could get better was by sharing their patient data nationwide. In its first year of data sharing, the Vermont

Oxford Network collected information submitted by 34 of the country's leading NICUs who thought that by banding together they could learn from each other and improve faster together. They were right. Today the Vermont Oxford Network stands out as one of the earliest and most substantive organizations dedicated to driving quality, safety, and continuous improvement in healthcare anywhere. Over 1,000 NICUs around the world now not only share their data—which now includes the records of well over 2 million infants—but participate in learning and improvement collaboratives that stretch across the globe.

Patients and their families are also more activated than at any time in history, but we still need even more activation. Every day, members of my family and yours make decisions about where to seek care based on what's important to them as consumers—things like how far away they are from a clinic, how challenging the hospital's parking lot is to navigate, the institution's reputation among friends and colleagues, and so on. These are important considerations, but unlike choosing a brand of laundry detergent, consumer-driven decisions about how, when, where, and with whom to seek healthcare carry with them measurably different outcomes, including potential harm or even death.

For years now, the Centers for Medicare and Medicaid Services have publicly reported measures of the quality of care provided by hospitals, including tracking whether every patient with a heart attack goes home with the appropriate aspirin prescription or whether any babies are delivered electively before 39 weeks without significant clinical justification. The same website also publicly reports even more striking outcomes, like how many heart attack patients die within 30 days of being discharged home.

There are real, measurable differences on metrics like these even among hospitals within the same community. Across the nation, over the course of a year, these differences add up to thousands of patients who live or die depending on which hospital they chose for care. Yet when my own mother needed elective surgery, she didn't even know HospitalCompare.gov existed, though I quickly brought her up to speed. She had talked to her friends and her neighbors and trusted that any hospital she picked would, of course, provide the highest quality care possible. This is plainly, simply, and unabashedly untrue.

In order to actually deliver care that agencies like the Centers for Medicare and Medicaid Services rank among the best in the nation, physicians, clinics, hospitals, and health systems must be committed to responding to mistakes using Just Culture. Their culture of safety must be firmly rooted in the board of directors, extend all the way through the leadership trunk, and out into every branch and leaf of front-line clinicians, and they must be committed to continuously improving everything they do even when they think they're already doing it well. They need to be appropriately transparent with patients, families, team members, and communities when they make mistakes, and then own finding and fixing systematic process errors that could have allowed the mistake to reach a patient.

Above all, they need to remember that every clinician is human, that humans are fallible and therefore will inevitably make mistakes. If they do, the center's leaders know it is their job to both teach and equip their teams to perform as best as they possibly can while surrounding them with enough layers of Swiss cheese to keep mistakes from falling through all the holes. I'm proud to get to do this now in my work both as a doctor and as a leader, and for such a personally and professionally fulfilling role, I have a 911 page mistake, a chief resident, a Cosmic Cantina burrito, and a legion of mentors like Drs. Karen Frush and Ronald Paulus who came thereafter to thank.

In closing out this chapter, I acknowledge it is possible that you've come to the terrifying realization that the next time you seek care, your doctor, nurse, or therapist may make a mistake in treating you. It's not only possible; at some point in your life, it's a mathematically foregone conclusion that at some point it will happen. So what can you do? You can act. Ask your providers about quality and patient safety, ask how it's measured and how it's practiced. Ask if the hospital and clinic teams you visit embrace the Just Culture model, whether they disclose mistakes and work with patients and families to recognize them, and whether they dedicate time and energy to finding and fixing the systematic root causes of errors to prevent them from reaching the next patient.

Research your doctors, your hospitals, your skilled nursing facilities, and your rehab centers, and read about their publicly reported outcomes. It's just like reading restaurant reviews on Yelp but with much greater potential impact. Learn what it takes to avoid the kinds of preventable harms you may experience when you're getting the care you need, be it a surgery (e.g., surgical site infections, falls, and catheter-associated urinary tract infections) or chemotherapy (central-line associated bloodstream infections), or just a routine checkup (medication errors). Make sure your providers are not only committed to but measurably and visibly doing all the evidence-based best practices you've read about, and ask about what you can do to participate in the safety process.

And for heaven's sake, don't let your doctor touch you without first washing his or her hands. Our profession has known better for 150 years.

– 6 –

Humanity, Technology, and the Future of Medicine

"Technology is nothing. What's important is that you have a faith in people, that they're basically good and smart, and if you give them tools, they'll do wonderful things with them. It's not the tools you have faith in—tools are just tools. They work, or they don't work. It's people you have faith in or not."

–Steve Jobs: *Rolling Stone Magazine*

At its core, healthcare has always been and will always be a uniquely human endeavor. Ask any nurse, therapist, paramedic, medical assistant, or doctor what brings her the most professional joy and you'll invariably hear one answer: people. More specifically, the greatest professional joys I've heard clinicians of every stripe describe derive most directly from spending meaningful time with their patients and spending meaningful time with their teams. The explanation is obvious. As clinicians, we are all called to healthcare to engage purposefully and completely with the most viscerally human characteristics of our existence—the tensions between strength and vulnerability, youth and aging, disease and wellbeing, life and death.

Yet 21st century healthcare pulls providers away from this core person-to-person interaction more than ever. In the nearly 20 years since I started medical school, I've seen the practice of medicine undergo a wholesale technological transformation. Take medical records as a simple example. I am 100% certain that today's second-year Duke medical students are much slower walkers than me. Why? Because the days of sprinting in your Danskos to get ahead of the white coat phalanx on rounds, pull down a door cabinet, and open a three-ring binder chart to the next blank page before the intern reaches the door ended nearly a decade ago. These newfangled medical students are also both blessed and cursed with electronic medical records that track and trend every aspect of a patient's health history, demanding hours of tedious, field-driven data entry but yielding treasure troves of new information. What used to require combing through binder upon binder of paper records by hand to learn about a patient's past medical history now takes just a few clicks. Health information technology has integrated itself into every aspect of the patient-provider relationship and will only become increasingly more pervasive as it improves and evolves.

This technological transformation played out one afternoon during my second year of NICU fellowship. Very early in my medical school days, I learned (like all good medical students) that when another clinician calls you and asks you to come see a baby—no matter why he's calling or what time it is—you get up and go. This simple axiom serves as well today as it did throughout medical school, internship, residency, and fellowship. As a fellow who lived by this principle, I'd developed a reputation as a doctor who wouldn't push back when a someone asked me to come to a baby's bedside.

This particular afternoon was fairly unremarkable. The Duke NICU was only moderately busy, and I'd just returned from the in-hospital Starbucks when a young clinician came running into the main provider work area. In a panic, she said, "Chris, Chris, I need you to come to Room 3 right now, this baby is apneic."

Apneic means not breathing, and not breathing is not good, so I flung my coffee cup behind the two tall computer monitors at the NICU fellow's workstation and took off with him down the hall. I expected to encounter a room filled with controlled chaos, a gaggle of people around an isolette with its plastic top ripped off, monitor alarms blaring, someone giving a bluish-looking baby positive pressure mask ventilation and someone else prepping an endotracheal tube and a ventilator. When I got to Room 3, though, I instead found four quiet isolettes in a quiet room with nothing apparently amiss. Puzzled, I looked at the clinician and asked, "I thought you said someone was apneic?" He looked at me equally puzzled, pointed to the monitor in bed-space C, and said, "This baby is apneic, look at the screen!"

My eyes darted from the infant's blanket-covered isolette to the flat-screen monitor above bed-space C, where I saw the usual physiologic tracings: a three-lead electrocardiogram monitor plotting out the continuous electrical activity of the baby's heart in a bright green glow, a light blue pulse oximeter displaying the baby's oxygen level and heart rate, a set of sterile white numbers declaring the infant's blood pressure to be normal, and a graceful yellow line tracing out the baby's sinusoidal breathing pattern. Everything seemed in order except the breathing rate, which, despite the gentle upward and downward deflecting yellow curve, read "0."

"See," he entreated, "he's apneic!"

I then noted that there were at least two things wrong. First, when babies really stop breathing, they also stop exchanging oxygen and carbon dioxide, meaning their pulse oximeter reading precipitously drops and ultimately so does their heart rate. This baby, despite having a breathing rate that read zero, had a totally normal heart rate and a blood oxygen level that was probably better than mine. Second, the infant's isolette was covered with a blanket so I couldn't actually see what was going on with the patient. Our NICU Division Chief and fellowship director Dr. Goldberg had flogged into our brains as fellows the need to physically look at a baby before believing a monitor, so I lifted the blanket. Sure enough, underneath and curled up in the fetal position was a comfortably breathing baby.

Relieved that we must have a faulty lead or monitor cable, I looked back to the clinician and said, "It's OK, she's breathing and the rest of her vitals are fine, must be a monitor issue." When I turned to go, I felt him grab my shoulder." "No," he said, this time more intensely, "the monitor says she's apneic, we can't just ignore it. We have to do something."

Totally confused at this point, I gestured to the rest of the monitor, explaining again that it was impossible for the baby girl to be both apneic and have a 100% oxygen saturation at the same time, at least not for very long. I then lifted the blanket again with the clinician next to me, cleaned my hands and wiped my stethoscope, and we both watched and listened to her breathe together. It took several more minutes before she believed both me and his own senses over the monitor reading. Despite more fussing with the monitor, its screen refused to truthfully report the infant's breathing rate until the charge nurse came by and helped change out the leads.

This story isn't meant in any way to belittle or shame the young clinician from that afternoon. His generation—one that's frankly not much younger than mine—has been taught to believe the story the technology tells them over the story their own eyes. The more intimately dependent we grow on technology—think about the radar alerts that come with some cars' backup cameras and tell you when you're getting too close to parking up a tree—the more we will come to question our own senses before we question a machine.

Truth be told, sometimes the technology is trying to show us something our eyes can't see. In healthcare today, data-driven algorithms can tell us that a patient who may clinically look well at a glance is actually at high risk of imminent decline. In these circumstances, believing your eyes over the machine's warning squanders an opportunity to intervene early and potentially prevent a patient from experiencing serious harm. Medicine's technological transformation has opened panoplies of new treatment doors to walk through with our patients, yet it's present focust also puts us at great risk of losing the raw humanity that has defined the practice of medicine since the days of Asclepius.

At times, technology may seem like the antithesis of humanity—it doesn't feel, doesn't connect, and too often pulls people into their screens and away from human contact rather than encouraging more of it. Liz Boehm—a good friend and leader in the patient, family, and clinician experience movement in healthcare—reminded me once that while technology-driven solutions are powerful, they all share one major weakness: "They can't see the humanity in the human in front of them." No technology can ease the despair of parents whose child you've just diagnosed with cancer, or of parents-to-be whose baby is being born weeks too early to survive. These human conversations require human compassion, and sharing human compassion is core to our humanity.

In a decade of practicing medicine, there is one patient with whom I've bonded over more of these human-to-human connections than any other. Ironically enough, our connection started with technology—technology, that is, and sports.

I met soon-to-be Dr. Stephen Kirchner when I was a pediatrics intern in the fall of 2008. I was on-service on the "Harris" team, the inpatient ward service that covered all pediatric hematology-oncology patients. In general, the service split more or less in half. One group of patients needed treatment for hematology problems like sickle cell anemia, a genetic condition where red blood cells aren't formed correctly. Instead of remaining nice round discs, under any kind of stress, they turn into something resembling a crescent moon. Patients with sickle cell anemia begin experiencing "pain crises" as early as infancy, which occur when sickled red blood cells accumulate in the ends of tiny blood vessels and can't get out, leading to intense pain and sometimes difficulty breathing. While such pain crises could get very serious, most of the time these patients were in and out of the hospital over the course of a few days.

The other half of the service were the oncology patients, whose hospital stays were more often measured in weeks to months. Some of the pediatric cancer patients would roll through our service fairly quickly, like those whose cancer was already diagnosed and under treatment but needed to be admitted for monitoring and antibiotics after having a fever, or others being admitted for a short course of chemotherapy and hydration during the middle stages of their multi-year treatment plan. Others wound up in the hospital on the Harris team for months on end, especially those who were newly diagnosed.

Stephen fell into the latter category. He'd been a completely healthy teenager, not that much younger than my brother, until one day he wasn't. He was bruising easily and tiring out while playing soccer much sooner than usual. A routine blood draw showed all three of his "cell lines" down, meaning his red blood cell count, white blood cell count, and platelet count were all below normal levels. Each of these cell lines are made from progenitor cells that usually live within our bone marrow. When all three levels are low, sometimes it means something else is crowding out the normal bone marrow cells so they can't make new blood cells. In kids (and more rarely in adults), that something else can be a blood cancer like leukemia.

After his blood draw that summer, Stephen was admitted to the Harris service to find out what was really going on. He underwent a barrage of additional testing and was ultimately diagnosed with a condition called myelodysplastic syndrome, a precursor to acute myeloid leukemia (AML). According to St. Jude's Children Research Hospital, only around 500 children in the United States are diagnosed with AML each year. While in the 1970s the survival rate for childhood AML was under 20%, when Stephen was diagnosed in 2008, the chances of survival had increased to over 50%[4]— a dramatic improvement to be sure, but still a 1 in 2

---

4   https://www.ncbi.nlm.nih.gov/pmc/articles/PMC3468705/

chance of dying. Diagnosis now in hand, Stephen faced a road to remission that would be exceptionally long, and he was only at the very beginning.

I was similarly at the beginning of a long road, though not one fraught with a 50% chance of death. I had started my intern year with two rotations that didn't require call, spending my first four-week block as a real doctor in the Duke Pediatric Same Day Clinic on Roxboro Road and my second block at the Durham Regional Hospital Special Care Nursery. My third block that fall would bring me into the wards of Duke Hospital on "Q4 call" for the first time, which would significantly ratchet up the intensity. "Q4 call" meant that throughout the month-long rotation, I'd start every fourth day in the hospital at 7 a.m., take sign-out from the previous call team, round on my own team's patients, admit new patients, then take sign-out around 5 p.m. from all the resident teams who got to go home. I'd then join one or two other residents to stay in-house all night, taking cross-cover calls, responding to emergencies, and admitting even more new patients. When 7 a.m. came again, I'd sign out, round on my own team of patients post-call, and go home ostensibly no later than 1 p.m., or around 32 hours after I'd come to the hospital the previous morning. All while taking care of around 20 kids with cancer during daytime hours and covering most of the nearly 100-patient pediatric ward service overnight.

While modern resident work-hour restrictions mean interns no longer take "Q4 call," at the time I did my internship, the Accreditation Council on Graduate Medical Education (the group that regulates resident and fellow training programs) was more lenient in its guidelines. To be clear, any restriction in work hours still made for a markedly different experience than the residency training programs of decades past, whose 24/7 in-house demand birthed the term "resident" in the first place. The generation of doctors who preceded me (and all those who preceded them) spent so much time at work they really didn't need an apartment and could have justifiably listed the hospital as their primary place of residence on their tax forms. By 2008, residency programs across America had to at least place basic guardrails around residents' hours, limiting trainees to taking in-house call no more frequently than every third night, working no more than 80 in-house hours per week averaged over four weeks and no more than 32 hours of work in the hospital in a row. We were also required to average one day off in seven, which yielded the new vocabulary term "Golden Weekend" when a resident somehow wound up with both a Saturday and a Sunday entirely off. Golden Weekends were exceptionally rare during my intern year, and I wound up working a lot of Sundays.

I began my month on the Harris service on Monday, August 25, 2008. While I can't remember exactly when I met Stephen during my Harris block, it must have been that first or second Sunday. That month on Harris was the first inpatient ward service I'd ever covered as a real doctor, and I was determined to know everything there was to know about my patients. Stephen became one of my patients, and we hit it off over SportsCenter.

For the uninitiated, SportsCenter is a show on the television network ESPN that essentially repeats the same one-hour collection of highlights from all of the major professional and college sports leagues over and over, stopping only to change anchors and update the stories in the evening with another day's worth of highlights. I had grown up watching SportsCenter, but with an intern's schedule, I didn't get to watch it much at the time and in Stephen I found a willing sports-watching partner. Soon after we met, I'd stop by his room after rounds and we'd watch the highlights, adding our own requisite color commentary from time to time. In the evenings on call nights that weren't too busy, I'd come by and eat my dinner in his room while he was eating his own and we'd catch the new SportsCenter highlights.

As late summer began its transition into early fall, the sport that most dominated the highlights on SportsCenter was the National Football League. I was always a baseball fan growing up and Stephen was an exceptional soccer player, but football was on so football is what we watched. It also happened that my brother was a sophomore in college that year, and to help us stay in touch, we'd decided to place a friendly bet on a random professional football game every weekend. Every Sunday thereafter for the next few months, I'd check in with Stephen, tell him the game of the week, and explain how my brother and I had made the bet. Something like: "I took the Steelers over the Packers at straight odds" or "Dolphins over the Jets on the betting line." Stephen in turn would reliably keep me updated as the day unfolded whenever I popped my head into his room, saying: "Dolphins are down by three in the second quarter" or "You're a total idiot, the Dolphins are getting creamed 38-3!" I'm fairly certain that Stephen's participation (especially as a minor) in this friendly family gambling each week didn't constitute a violation of federal or state law, but if it did, I'm hopeful any government officials who happen to be reading this will have mercy on me.

One weekend later in the year, our football bonding did go a bit too far. I'd rotated off the Harris team by that point, but Stephen was still in the middle of his induction chemotherapy regimen and had moved down the hall on the pediatric ward into the vaunted room 5131. Not all in-patient rooms on the Duke Hospital wards are created equal—at least at the time, I remember most being just large enough to fit a hospital bed, a bathroom, and a couch. Stephen had started his long stay in one of those rooms—something like room 5127 if memory serves. However, as soon as it became clear he'd need to stay in the hospital for months to complete his initial treatment pathway, the team started looking to get him and his family into one of the unit's handful of larger, long-term rooms.

Room 5131 (again, at least as I remember it) is huge. It's more than twice the size of any other room on the unit, has two entry doors, big exterior windows, and was immediately to the right of the main nursing station. Relative to everything else on the pediatric unit, and frankly in the entire hospital, it felt gigantic. However, giving a teenager and a 27-year-old guy this kind of space in the middle of football season meant one thing—we had to play Nerf ball.

Pediatric teams (especially a group known as "Child Life") work incredibly hard to bring as many "normal" aspects of life into the hospital as possible for pediatric cancer patients. For a teenage kid, Nerf balls definitely count as a normal aspect of life, so we had access to them in abundance. What we hadn't considered were the challenges involved in safely throwing around a Nerf ball when your platelet count is very, very low.

Platelets are small fragments of cells that originate from bone marrow precursors and course through every human's bloodstream. Platelets are incredibly useful, helping our blood clot whenever we get a cut.

They're also generally incredibly numerous, with a normal platelet count hovering in the range of 250,000 platelets per microliter of blood. An average-size human has around 5.5 liters of blood, yielding on the order of 1.5 trillion platelets. However, when you're receiving induction chemotherapy for AML, the precursor cells that live in the bone marrow and make things like platelets, red blood cells, and white blood cells, are wiped out along with the cancerous leukemia cells lurking there as well. While we can give patients transfusions of red blood cells and platelets, each individual blood transfusion carries some risk as does the cumulative number of transfusions a patient receives over the course of their cancer treatment. Thus, best practice in pediatric oncology demands that we generally wait to transfuse platelets into childhood cancer patients' blood until their levels are much lower than normal.

Which brings us back to our Nerf ball game that late fall weekend. That day I'd finished rounding on an in-patient general pediatrics service, and had come by to spend whatever part of the afternoon my pager would allow to watch our game of the week and throw around the Nerf ball. Since Stephen wasn't my direct patient anymore, I didn't know what his "counts" were, but his platelets were apparently low. Not just a little low—extremely low, around 20 times lower than normal and just above the level at which he'd need a transfusion.

Oblivious to the potential hazards, we'd turned on the game and were throwing the ball around when Stephen reared his right arm back to really whip one at me. As he cocked his arm, he proceeded to whack his elbow against the hard-plastic edge of his bed. Under normal circumstances, the response from any male member of the human race to such a whack would be "Owww!"

This would quickly be followed by the development of a small bruise, and an immediate return to throwing the ball hard enough to both dull the pain and ensure the other guy winds up with at least as big a bruise when he tries to catch it. Ours, however, were not normal circumstances. With his platelet count in the cellar, Stephen's bruise immediately expanded like one of those "Magic Grow" sponge animals that octuple in size in a matter of seconds after you drop them in water.

Dismayed by the immediacy of our need to return from the "normal" world back to the world of the pediatric cancer ward, we gave his oncology team a call. They deftly treated his elbow and addressed his platelet count so he wouldn't wind up with a permanently elephantine arm. Thankfully, no long-term harm was done, but I was terrified of running into his attending pediatric oncologist or his primary pediatric oncology fellow from that point on.

As the year wore on, Stephen's journey with AML continued as did my own journey in residency. Stephen was the first patient I really got to know as a person—I got to know his family, where they were from, what he liked and didn't like, and what school was like for him. In turn, I told him about my own life, about getting married, about medical school, and about being a doctor. We both talked about what we "wanted to be when we grew up." And we spent a long, long time talking about sports. Some days I'd come by and find him sleeping, so I talked to his mother, his father, or his grandparents and I got to know both about Stephen through their eyes and a little about their own lives. At Christmas that year, while I was again covering the Harris team a week before my daughter's birth, his family gave me a beautiful wooden ornament of a doctor in his white coat. I keep the ornament in my office to this day, and it remains the one and only gift I've ever accepted from a patient.

In late 2008, Stephen's oncology team decided his best opportunity to beat cancer would require him to go through the grueling bone marrow transplant process. The process at the time unfolded inside a locked, hermetically sealed bone marrow transplant unit on Duke Hospital's fifth floor, with a team of doctors and other caregivers that did not include residents. I still came by to visit him, now having to brave the bone marrow unit's lengthy entrance procedure and requirement for hazmat-like donning of personal protective equipment just to get through its multiple locked doors. Once he made it through the initial transplant, I also got to see him from time to time as an outpatient in the pediatric oncology clinic. I remember once he needed treatment for something called graft-versus-host disease, a condition where donor white blood cells from the bone marrow transplant attack the recipient's organs until the cells are either wiped out or reconditioned. I've heard pediatric oncologists say a little graft-versus-host disease is at least a sign that the transplant is taking root, and in Stephen's case it thankfully did. By the time I finished residency and went on to NICU fellowship, he had also completed his treatment and returned home to finish high school.

Then on a random March day in 2013, I got an email out of the blue from Stephen. It came from an "@duke.edu" email address, and I was amazed to learn that not only had Stephen finished high school but was now an undergraduate student at Duke and doing research in the hospital. We caught up for the first time in years on campus, and have stayed in touch ever since. Stephen is now a third-year MD/PhD student at Duke, smar er than I'll ever hope to be, and at the time I wrot this chapter totally smashing his first round of United States Medical Licensing Examination Step exams and preparing for his years in the lab. It's been the privilege of a lifetime as a pediatrician to be able to see one of my patients beat AML, beat high school, beat college, and now beat medical school. For what's now become the possibility of a new lifelong connection—one of life's rarest and most precious gifts—I have the intersection of technology and humanity to thank.

This begs the question—could technology actually help return some humanity to healthcare? I truly believe it can, and my experience with Stephen highlights how. Imagine stripping away all of the tasks involved in the delivery of healthcare that do not absolutely require humans to perform. All that remains would be the raw humanity ingrained in person-to-person interactions. While forming a connection with a patient over nationally televised professional football is perhaps a simplistic example, better technology can both enable and expand our humanity by facilitating more of the right kinds of human-to-human contacts.

One of the most valuable lessons I learned in training was how to differentiate "sick" from "not sick" and "toxic" from "not toxic." It's a skill that requires seeing thousands of patients one by one, each with a unique constellation of symptoms, all taking slightly different trajectories in the courses of their illness. Over time, as a doctor's brain adds more and more examples of patients with a particular disease to his collective experience, clear patterns emerge. With each new patient I add another set of observations to my mental library, clarifying the tiny variations in history, symptoms, physical exam, and laboratory findings that could help predict which patients may take which course.

As an intern on the general pediatrics ward, one of the clearest examples of this kind of pattern recognition involved patients with severe asthma attacks. Children with asthma who need to be hospitalized are without question "sick." I'd see them first in clinic or in the emergency department, their parents administering medications to them through inhalers at home at least every four hours. Despite the maximum home treatment regimen, these patients would present for care often barely clinging to stable breathing rates and oxygen levels. They would be breathing faster than normal, and when I listened to their lungs, I could hear the unmistakable "wheezing" associated with asthma when they breathed both in and out. Sometimes parts of their lungs would be so constricted I couldn't hear air moving at all.

When I say these patients were "sick," I mean there was a reasonable enough chance that they would get worse before they got better and therefore I couldn't send them home. As a general pediatrics ward intern, getting a call from the emergency department for "a kid with asthma who looks sick" meant a night of constant observation to be sure the child wouldn't become "toxic." On nights like those, I'd circle the ward like a hawk checking room by room to monitor vital signs and listen to breath sounds to find out if I could hear air moving throughout the lungs and, if so, how bad the wheezing sounded. I'd watch especially closely if the child had fallen asleep to see how hard he or she had to work to breathe while completely at rest. The vast majority of these patients would turn the corner from "sick" to "not sick" within hours to days, but a small minority would advance to looking "toxic" even with the best treatments we had to offer.

When a patient looks "toxic," it means that even at a glance you know that without some kind of rapid intervention they are at high risk of complete physiologic collapse. As I later learned in NICU fellowship, both children with asthma and newborns with respiratory distress syndrome display many of the same concerning symptoms as they begin the descent from "sick" to "toxic." Kids have an amazing capacity to breathe way faster than adults and for a much longer period of time before tiring out. That said, once children—newborn or otherwise—start to tire out, they are at incredibly high risk of quickly falling apart.

I've witnessed both children with asthma and newborns with respiratory distress syndrome go from breathing fast on their own—but no longer fast enough to maintain good oxygen and carbon dioxide exchange— to requiring 100% oxygen and the maximum amount of high-frequency ventilator support we can provide just to return their oxygen and carbon dioxide levels to baseline. These kids look "toxic," and our job as doctors is to recognize the evolving pattern from "sick" to "toxic" as early as possible, prevent the descent if we are able, and treat it as aggressively as modern medicine allows.

The first child I remember identifying as "toxic" was an infant with respiratory distress who I had admitted to the hospital during my "acting internship" rotation as a fourth-year medical student. Alan* was a former preemie who at that point was maybe 11 months old and had contracted a condition called bronchiolitis caused by respiratory syncytial virus (RSV). For adults and most kids, RSV just causes a bad cold. However, for very young babies, former preemies, and anyone with underlying lung problems, RSV can lead to bronchiolitis, a condition where the infecting virus causes shedding of the cellular linings inside the lung's small-to-medium airways called bronchioles. This viral shedding leads to a buildup of mucus-laden tissue that intermittently blocks any air from passing through the bronchioles. Children with RSV bronchiolitis have a classic "crackle and wheeze" noise when you listen to their breath sounds and often need to work very hard to breathe. The condition lasts for days until the shedding finally stops and patients can clear out the blockages through lots and lots of coughing.

Alan was admitted to the hospital early in the course of his illness and he was the first child I'd ever cared for with RSV bronchiolitis. I remember watching how fast he was breathing and how hard the muscles in between his ribs and under his chin were pulling to support his weakening diaphragm. My resident said all of this was to be expected with RSV at this point in Alan's course, but that we needed to watch him very closely because no baby can keep up that amount of work just to breathe forever without needing help. Unfortunately, we don't have many options to treat or change the course of RSV, so instead we watch, wait, supplement the room air these children breathe with extra oxygen, and monitor very closely as the patient's own immune system does most of the work.

I was walking through the pediatric ward late in the evening after we'd admitted Alan to our service and stopped by his room to make sure he was OK. He wasn't. Even a medical student could tell the glassy look in his eyes wasn't normal, and he had one of the telltale signs of a child who has worked too hard to breathe for too long and was beginning to tire out. Infants with

RSV bronchiolitis who are working to breathe first begin using the muscles in between their ribs and flare out their nostrils to generate the extra force needed to overcome the extra resistance. Next, they start pulling hard on their neck muscles, which at its most extreme makes a patient look almost like one of those weird expandable-neck spitting dinosaurs from Jurassic Park. When all of these efforts fail, infants start to "see-saw" their chests up and down, their bellies protruding out while their breast bones suck down. Finally, when infants are beginning to tire out but before they totally collapse, you can see their breastbone switch from moving back and forth like a see-saw to moving listlessly up and down. That's what a glassy-eyed Alan looked like when I walked by his room that night.

Noticing his glazed stare from the hallway, I darted into his room and glanced first at his monitor. It showed a fast heart rate, a slow breathing rate, and an oxygen level that was barely clinging to 90%. His eyes were dull, his pupils barely fixed on my face, and his breastbone was unmistakably moving up and down instead of back and forth. I immediately ran out the door and called for help from the rapid response team. Within seconds a deluge of more senior staff, from residents to respiratory therapists to the pediatric intensive care team, came running to the room and whisked Alan to a higher level of care. He wound up doing just fine after receiving more intense support, returned to our service within a day or so, and went home shortly thereafter. However, for the rest of my days, I will never forget that first experience watching a patient take the quick tumble from "sick" to "toxic."

Once a doctor learns to differentiate "sick" from "not sick" and "toxic" from "not toxic," it's like wearing glasses for the first time. While the corrective lenses are never perfect—any patient on any day can fool a doctor by looking and sounding fine while being on the verge of imminent disaster—the prescription gets just a little bit better with every patient you see. But even the best glasses won't bend the laws of physics to let you see a hundred patients on a pediatric ward service or 68 critically ill NICU babies all at once. This leaves even the best doctors with the most powerful and finely tuned lenses always a step behind.

Yet thankfully it no longer has to be this way. We live in an era of augmented intelligence, where our smartphones use intelligent algorithms to guess where we want to go or what we want to say next. Similarly, clinicians can partner with data science wizards to produce clinical computer algorithms trained on billions of data points. These algorithms comb the electronic medical record to train on past patients' trajectories in the same way clinicians are trained, honing the lenses of their own prescription glasses patient by patient by the millions. Used in real time, these models can predict impending doom by aggregating every bit of information produced by network-connected vital signs monitors and anything documented in an electronic medical record to predict looming potential for disaster before it happens. I've personally seen at least two such systems in use today, one that specifically tracks the beat-to-beat variability of every infant's heart rate in a NICU and another that collates data points from nursing assessments, vital signs, and laboratory values for patients across an entire hospital.

As systems like these become increasingly perfected, technology will enable us to extend the lenses of individual clinicians over hundreds, if not thousands, of patients at once. Like a sheepdog continually circling its herd, technology like this offers doctors a better chance to use our human training, experience, and intuition to intervene and prevent a patient's descent from well to sick or from sick to toxic earlier and for more people than ever. I was lucky to have seen Alan when I did, before a precipitous drop in his oxygen levels would have sent his monitor alarms into maximum-squeal mode and beckoned the team running into his room for a potential code situation. While the great 1930s New York Yankees pitcher Lefty Gomez once said, "I'd rather be lucky than good"—with increasingly well-tuned healthcare technology, I'm hopeful we can get from "good" to "better" with less reliance on luck.

It is perhaps our nature that we often focus on what makes the practice of medicine something that needs fixing. That's OK, because as with any human endeavor we will never reach perfection and thus have an endless number of opportunities to improve. However, sometimes our focus on what's wrong makes us forget about all that's right, the things that make the United States a beacon that lights the world of medicine as brightly as it lights the world at large. Perhaps more powerfully than anywhere else on earth, in America liberty begets freedom—freedom of thought, freedom of action, and freedom to imagine a world beyond that which now exists. Such freedoms have thus made perpetual technological innovation central to the story of American medicine for centuries.

In the early 1950s, an American doctor named Robert Guthrie pioneered the concept of universal newborn screening. He had perfected a fast, cheap way to test newborn babies for phenylketonuria (PKU), a condition caused by the inability of a baby's body to break down the amino acid phenylalanine. As a result, chemicals called "toxic metabolites" build up inside the brain of an infant with PKU leading to permanent developmental delay. This outcome, however, is 100% preventable if the condition is identified early and the baby's diet is modified to avoid significant amounts of phenylalanine. Dr. Guthrie's PKU test has not only saved thousands of babies from a lifetime of unremitting seizures and profound developmental challenges, but his universal newborn screening idea has expanded to many more conditions. In North Carolina in 2018, the state performs tests for no less than 37 separate conditions on a single blood-spot card, ranging from PKU to congenital adrenal hyperplasia to "Long-Chain L-3 Hydroxyacyl-CoA Dehydrogenase Deficiency."

Sixty years after Dr. Guthrie's PKU test revolutionized medicine and many revisions later, I was fortunate to use North Carolina's universal newborn screening as an intern to diagnose an infant with a condition four times rarer than PKU. It's a condition that's totally asymptomatic until a mild viral infection triggers a terrifying cascade of symptoms including a plummeting blood sugar, vomiting, and seizures that, left untreated, could lead to death. Instead, having caught the condition on a newborn screen, my general pediatrics attending and I educated the infant's parents about the condition and connected them to an expert in genetics and metabolics well before their daughter ever got sick. She's now in grade school and has a chance to live a totally normal life.

I keep two of my most prized medical possessions on a bookshelf in my office at home. The first, *Combe's Physiology*, is an 1843 edition of a text by Andrew Combe, MD, "Physician Extraordinaire to the Queen in Scotland and Consulting Physician to the King and Queen of the Belgians." The title page takes care to note that six woodcuts appear in this seventh edition of a book whose full title takes several lines to complete:

The Principles of Physiology
applied to the
Preservation of Health
and to the improvement of
Physical and Medical Education

The second book is simply titled *Physician's Handbook* and is the eighth edition of a manuscript by Lange Medical Publications published in 1954.

Leafing through these texts offers a window into the world of technology and innovation in medicine over the last 200 years. It also demonstrates why keeping pace with advances in medicine today is not just a little harder than it was for physicians in the days of Oliver Wendell Holmes Sr. It is in truth exponentially harder, requiring enough energy and effort that it challenges the time needed to make the fundamental, human-to-human core interactions with patients that define the practice of medicine itself.

Take for example the management of infectious diseases. In *Combes Physiology*—written before either Pasteur or Semmelweis and three years after Britain began providing free smallpox vaccination using Jenner's cowpox inoculation without any clue how it worked—the word "infection" doesn't even appear in the Index. Rather, Chapter X "Application of the Preceding Principles" speaks to what the author believed to be *"the real origin of bad health."* There were, in fact, thought to be three such "origins" (pages 308-309):

"First, as having no necessary connexion with our conduct, but as being the result of circumstances entirely beyond our knowledge and control, and sent by a superintending Providence, not to urge us to more rational care, but to soften our hearts and warn us from sin. Secondly, as the result of accident alone or of external influencers which we can appreciate, but from which it is impossible to withdraw ourselves. Thirdly, as, in every instance, the result of the direct infringement of one or more of the laws or conditions decreed by the Creator to be essential to the well-being and activity of every bodily organ, and the knowledge and observance of which are, to a great extent, within our power."

By the 1950s, physician-scientists had clarified many of the "circumstances" previously thought to be "entirely beyond our knowledge and control" including the concept of infectious diseases. So much so that eight whole pages of *Physician's Handbook* were devoted to "Chemotherapeutic and Antibiotic Agents" and page 380 even included a table of which diseases the seven available antibiotics were most suitable to treat.

In contrast, as of October 2018, Wikipedia's "List of Antibiotics" page counts no fewer than 148 different drugs while its "List of Antivirals" includes 87 medications in a section that the *Physician's Handbook* doesn't speak to at all. This, of course, is because the first antiviral (Acyclovir) wasn't even developed until 1977. The World Health Organization's 2013 *Critically important antimicrobials for human medicine* report runs to 31 pages and lists more classes of antibiotics than the *Physician's Handbook* table included actual drugs. Finally, the *Journal of Infectious Diseases*, which began as a quarterly publication in 1904 and is now published biweekly, yields over 2,000 pages of new infection-related science each year. And that's just one journal.

NICU medicine provides another remarkable example. While *Combes* doesn't devote much copy to the care of newborns, it does celebrate the utility of fresh air and country living as a public health intervention to reduce infant mortality, a critical public health measure tracking death within the first year of life. From page 312:

"A hundred years ago [the mid 18th century], when the pauper infants of London were received and brought up in the workhouses, amid impure air, crowding, and want of proper food, not above one in twenty-four lived to be a year old; so that out of 2800 annually received into them 2690 died. But when the conditions of health came to be a little better understood, and an act of Parliament was obtained obliging the parish officers to send the infants to nurse in the country, this frightful mortality was reduced to 450 instead of 2600!"

While a reduction in infant mortality from 96.1% to 16.1% is astonishingly successful, by the time *Physician's Handbook* was published 100 years later, infant mortality in the United States was down to 2.6% and still only four whole pages of the book were devoted to newborn care under "Infant Feeding." These included a table of the appropriate proportions of Karo syrup, water, and evaporated milk to mix when making "formulae for Artificial Feeding." Dr. Virginia Apgar's APGAR score, developed one year earlier in 1953, isn't mentioned at all and the American Board of Pediatrics wouldn't offer the first board certification exam in neonatology until 1974.

Since then, the *Journal of Perinatology*—again, only one of many peer-reviewed journals specific to newborn medicine and only published in its current form since 1984—now produces over 1,000 pages of material each year related to the care of high-risk mothers and premature newborns. By 2016, America's infant mortality rate had inched even further down to 0.6% while offering many extremely premature infants—who wouldn't have even been considered "live births" in the 1840s or 1950s—a chance at survival.

In my lifetime alone, estimates of the doubling time of medical knowledge have dropped from every eight years in the 1980s to a projected 73 days by 2020. If this holds true, by the time a medical student in the entering class of 2020 graduates in 2024, she will have watched the world's complement of knowable medical information increase nearly 1,000,000 times (or 20 doublings over four years). What's more, remember she's already starting from a place much different than Holmes or even me. If we got from "fresh air" to penicillin with a doubling time measured in centuries, and from simply measuring an APGAR score to saving more than half of 24-week preemies with a doubling time measured in decades, it is literally impossible to imagine where we will be a decade from now with doubling times measured in days.

Which once again brings us back to Stephen, the MD/PhD student. Stephen's commitment to research is emblematic of the driving force behind this rapidly advancing doubling time. As you read these lines, he's hard at work in a laboratory somewhere on the Duke University campus completing his PhD research before returning to the wards to finish medical school. Cancer-free for nearly a decade, he is a smart, strong, and energetic young man dedicating his career to the advancement of the same field that saved his own life. Indeed, in the annals of medical history, both his career and mine will likely be graded most heavily on our contributions to the understanding and treatment of disease and our efforts to promote and even accelerate medicine's continued technological advancement.

Yet it is the personal practice of medicine, not his contributions to science, that enable him to form the same human-to-human connection with individual patients that I was fortunate to fashion with him. While perhaps not measured in journal articles or academic promotions, I believe this core of humanity that has typified all of medicine for millennia is the far greater measure of our career success. By succeeding in the former, we enable doctors to be better at the latter, spending more time at their patient's bedsides and simply being human.

– 7 –

Never Give Up

"Surely from this period of ten months this is the lesson: never give in, never give in, *never, never, never, never give in; nothing, great or small, large or petty*—never give in except to convictions of honour and good sense. Never yield to force; never yield to the apparently overwhelming might of the enemy."

–Sir Winston Churchill: *Remarks at Harrow School*

I'd be dishonest if I didn't admit where the title of this chapter really comes from. A few years ago, my kids went totally nuts over *The Peanuts Movie*, a 21st century story involving Charles Schulz's classic Charlie Brown crew. We watched it so many times that the entire family could quote most of the film's dialogue word for word. It's a cute movie, and in my 6-year-old's favorite part, Snoopy is sitting atop his doghouse with a typewriter. He's writing a novel about his dauntless alter ego, a daring pilot named the Flying Ace, and imagines a scene where the Flying Ace's fair maiden Fifi is taken captive by the treacherous Red Baron. The camera pans out into something like a dream sequence, and we see Snoopy imagine the Flying Ace and his Sopwith Camel crash to the ground as the Red Baron's zeppelin flies off with Fifi in tow.

The movie then snaps back to Snoopy who, with a determined look, returns to his typewriter and begins the next chapter. He hammers at the keyboard while a narrator (who sounds suspiciously like Linus) reads the words:

Chapter Seven: Never Give Up!

"The Flying Ace knew he could never give up on her. He could never give up on himself. He repaired his plane and flew back to the aerodrome. Then he gathered his own squadron of Sopwith Camel planes. They took off in the darkness of night, headed for the ocean…"

Whether you've seen the movie or not, you of course already know the rest. Snoopy rescues Fifi from the Red Baron, the Allies win the war, and all is once again right with the world. It's the sweetest kind of triumph because, in order to taste it, the hero must first stare down the precipice of failure and choose to stay in the fight. While simplified for an animated children's movie, Snoopy's story is no less an analogy for the kinds of triumphs I've found most deeply fulfilling in the practice of medicine—those that require never giving up.

Like Snoopy, I am also a total flight junkie. While there were many things that convinced me to sign up for NICU fellowship, one of the biggest was the opportunity to join Duke's LifeFlight crews on helicopter transports all over the state. I'd never flown in a helicopter before I went to medical school, but it seemed like something I'd love if I ever had the chance. I was totally right.

In the early 2000s, the pilot and two critical care transport nurses on Duke's LifeFlight crew only took up three of the helicopter's four seats, meaning they could occasionally take a ride-along medical student. As a first-year medical student, I got to join the team for just one trip—a quick flight to somewhere in the eastern part of North Carolina to pick up a trauma patient and then back to Duke—but from that point on I was hooked.

At Duke, NICU fellows were expected to hop onboard with the LifeFlight team for either ground or air transports for two types of babies: those who were extremely premature and those who were extremely sick. For the former, we went along because we were some of the most experienced intubators of extraordinarily tiny windpipes. For the latter, we went both to help perform specialized NICU procedures and to be able to make the moment-to-moment decisions during neonatal resuscitation in person rather than over the phone a hundred miles away. While my wife was never a fan of my late-night text messages that usually said something like "Lifting off for Fayetteville—Love you," the flights I took with Duke's LifeFlight helicopter team will forever be among my most treasured memories in clinical practice. For the most part, these transports were fairly standard fare—fly into a small hospital where we'd be welcomed like the cavalry, pick up the baby, and fly home—but there is one trip that was decidedly different.

I was in the middle of fellowship when the call came through. It was from a NICU in another part of North Carolina, and they had a baby who just wasn't responding to any of their treatments. Her name was Ashanti*, and within minutes of her birth, her NICU team had her intubated on 100% oxygen with full ventilator support and high doses of blood pressure medications and antibiotics. None of it was working, and with her oxygen levels hovering dangerously below normal on such maximal support, the team wanted to transfer her to a center that could rapidly place her on something called "ECMO."

ECMO is "never give up" incarnate. The abbreviation stands for extracorporeal membranous oxygenation which, in the simplest terms, is a treatment that effectively takes over a patient's entire cardiovascular and respiratory systems. There are technically two kinds of ECMO—the first is VV, or venovenous ECMO, which acts essentially like an external lung. The second is VA, or venoarterial ECMO, which acts as both an external lung and an external heart.

VV-ECMO is used in circumstances where a patient's lungs are temporarily unable to function but expected to recover. In newborns, the classic VV-ECMO case is a baby with such severe pneumonia at birth that even the highest ventilation settings won't allow her lungs to exchange oxygen and carbon dioxide. When this happens, as long as the NICU team believes her lungs have a good chance of recovering within days to a few weeks, they can consider placing her on VV-ECMO until her lungs start doing the work of gas exchange again on their own.

VA-ECMO is a step even further up in criticality, as it's primarily used when a patient's heart or her heart and lungs are temporarily unable to function. In older children, a condition called viral myocarditis would be a classic case for VA-ECMO where—in exceptionally rare cases—common viruses that usually trigger mild cold symptoms can winnow through the bloodstream to infect a patient's heart. When this happens, the infecting virus can weaken the heart muscle, which makes it floppy. Floppy hearts don't generate much force, so the patient's blood pressure drops so dangerously low that medication alone can't fix it. Under these circumstances, VA-ECMO may be the only option to take over for the patient's own heart and lungs until the immune system wins its battle against the virus and the heart muscle recovers its strength.

In either case, I believe ECMO to be the most intense form of treatment medicine has to offer—a lifeline that, while a patient's chances of dying during treatment remains very high, can offer hope when there is no other option. And what an option it is. The pediatric cardiovascular surgeons first sedate the baby, give her pain medications, and administer a drug that temporarily paralyzes her so she won't move during the cannulation procedure. After a surgical time-out, the surgeons then very carefully use a scalpel, blunt forceps, and other tiny specialized tools to dissect away the skin of her neck and find the carotid artery and the internal jugular vein.

Having located their target, once the enormous pump machine sitting next to the baby's bed is fully primed with blood, they place one large catheter (also called a cannula) into the artery and another into the vein. The perfusionist team then turns on the pump and within seconds the infant's oxygen level and blood pressure normalize. It sounds simple, yet imagine the infant's entire blood supply now traveling out of her body through the cannula in her jugular vein, coursing through the ECMO membrane where oxygen and carbon dioxide are exchanged, and then pumping back into her body through the artery's cannula. Incredible doesn't even begin to describe it.

After hearing the story from the outside hospital, our NICU team thought Ashanti would likely need to immediately proceed onto VA-ECMO as both her oxygen levels and her blood pressure were low and unresponsive to anything they had thrown at her. She had a very high likelihood of dying before we even arrived—if she was still alive when we landed, we were by no means then guaranteed the chance to leave. Were we to be lucky enough to get her out of the outside hospital NICU, into the helicopter, and back to Duke, our instructions were to go straight to the pediatric cardiac intensive care unit where the pediatric cardiovascular surgeons and an entire operating room team would be waiting to begin the cannulation procedure. With all this in mind, we decided to take the risk and try the transport. My NICU attending handed me a small IV bag of epinephrine and my stethoscope, gave me a solid pat on both shoulders, and sent me on my way to meet LifeFlight on the roof.

After perhaps a 45-minute flight, we landed with an urgent "thump" on the outside hospital's helipad. Their security team escorted us into the NICU where I found exactly what I'd expected. Already sedated and paralyzed and under the bright lights of her warmer bed was Ashanti, a roughly 7-pound newborn with umbilical lines in place and several intravenous pumps of fluid and medications running. She was intubated and on maximum high-frequency ventilator settings, which presented a significant challenge as we would have to transport her on a regular ventilator. High-frequency ventilators deliver 7-10 tiny breaths per second, oscillating like a pulsar and sounding something like a drumroll. As a result, the physics of high-frequency ventilation allow us to deliver newborns at much higher pressures than regular ventilators can safely provide without risking serious complications. We had to find a way to stabilize Ashanti on our regular transport ventilator and fix her blood pressure at least long enough to get her back to Duke and into the pediatric cardiac intensive care unit to begin her ECMO course.

On the transport team with me that day were two incredibly experienced critical care transport nurses, both of whom had received additional special training to perform this kind of high-wire neonatal intensive care in the field and in the air. We spent hours together at her bedside using every trick we knew to get Ashanti stable enough to have a window to fly back to Durham. We gave her fluid boluses, epinephrine, prostaglandins, more sedation, and more fluid. We tweaked her ventilator settings, moving the pressures up and down and calibrating even the most minor controls in an effort to find the perfect balance. By the end of hour four, all three of us were sweating both mentally and physically and the pilot was beginning to run up against the limit of his Federal Aviation Administration-mandated shift end-time. Finally, after one last round of epinephrine and a minor, seemingly insignificant adjustment in her ventilator settings, Ashanti's oxygen level rose just above 90% and her blood pressure leveled. The crew and I looked at each other and decided it was now or never.

The lead transport nurse radioed out to the pilot, telling him to fire up the rotors so we could leave immediately upon loading the stretcher-bound isolette in the back of the helicopter. With three pairs of hands, we moved Ashanti from her warmer bed into the transport isolette, using a level of extreme caution that "careful" doesn't even begin to approach. Miraculously, her vital signs remained the same, just stable enough for transport but nowhere near stable enough to breathe a sigh of relief. We then rolled out of the NICU, through the hall, out the door and into the back of the helicopter in record time. There wasn't room in the back of the LifeFlight helicopter for the NICU fellow to sit with the crew, so I hopped into my perch up front next to the pilot. Throughout the flight, the lead nurse read off Ashanti's mean arterial blood pressure and oxygen saturation every minute or so over our helmet communications system and I prayed our interventions would keep her stable.

LifeFlight helicopters generally have a top speed somewhere in the range of 150 MPH. That said, I am convinced we broke the sound barrier that night on our way back to Duke. We screamed across North Carolina at low altitude to preserve the cabin's barometric pressure and oxygen tension, hitting each bank turn along the flight path home like a rollercoaster reaching its highest peak. Within what felt like barely a few minutes, we landed back on the roof of Duke Hospital in the pitch black of night, the surrounding university campus lit by the Duke Chapel's spiritual glow contrasted against the hospital roof's bright fluorescent blaze. With Ashanti's window of relative stability just beginning to close, we hustled into the elevator, rode down to the fifth floor, and broke through the doors into the pediatric cardiac intensive care unit. I handed off her care to the awaiting squadron of no fewer than 10 doctors and the entire operating room team, all prepared to take her straight onto VA-ECMO.

Then, just as the pediatric cardiothoracic surgery team began opening the trays needed to prepare for ECMO cannulation, the pediatric cardiologist moved in to repeat her echocardiogram one last time. She had already had several echocardiograms (heart ultrasounds) performed at the outside hospital's NICU before her transport, but he wanted to look once more for himself to confirm there was no structural heart problem that could be causing all of Ashanti's problems. Incredibly, as he moved the probe over the familiar-looking structures inside the baby's heart, he immediately saw the problem. One of Ashanti's heart valves was totally stuck, looking less like an oscillating stopcock than a tiny peace sign carved into cement. The stuck valve meant blood couldn't pass through that portion of her heart at all, and that instead of going straight onto ECMO, Ashanti needed the cardiologist to perform an emergency bedside cardiac catheterization procedure to save her life. He did—with a mammoth audience of doctors, nurses, techs, and the entire pediatric cardiothoracic surgery team watching each move—and she survived. She still needed complex surgery in the days thereafter, but ultimately did well and came to spend time with us in the NICU convalescing before going home a few weeks after her very eventful birth.

Ashanti's story is just one example of many that convince me we can choose to not give up. I can't explain why that last tiny tweak gave us a window of stability, why that window lasted just long enough to get her back to Duke, or why the cardiologist just happened to take that last echocardiogram. All I know is that she didn't give up, so neither did we.

The "never give up" maxim has held as true for me outside of medicine as it has within, a lesson I relearned as recently as this fall when I completed my first Ironman. For the uninitiated, an Ironman is a very, very, very long race composed of the three disciplines in triathlon. According to triathlon folklore (and Wikipedia), the Ironman's ridiculous distances descend from combining three 1970s-era Hawaiian races—the 2.4-mile Waikiki Roughwater Swim, a 115-mile Oahu bike race, and the Honolulu Marathon—into one massive race. When in 1978 the first competitors shaved 3 miles off the original bike race's course to create an easier transition zone from swim to bike and bike to run, the now iconic "Swim 2.4 miles! Bike 112 miles! Run 26.2 miles! Brag for the rest of your life!" ethos of Ironman Triathlon was born.

Back in 2003, I had actually volunteered as a first-year medical student at the Blue Devil Ironman. As exhausted and elated triathletes crossed the finish line, I worked the medical tent and escorted those who were dehydrated, hyponatremic, or obviously suffering from altered mental status into the tent for fluids. I remember thinking a person would have to suffer from significantly altered mental status at baseline just to sign up for such insanity, much less complete one. It turned out I was totally right.

I had trained for my race—Ironman Louisville on October 14, 2018—for over a year, having barely finished a half-distance Ironman 70.3 race alive in 2017. Shortly after crossing the line in Raleigh that summer, profoundly dehydrated and unable to stand without help, I was rescued by my wife, who parked me in a wheelchair and whisked me into the medical tent as a patient this time for intravenous fluids and something called "salted Gatorade." It tastes just as bad as it sounds. Midway through the second liter of intravenous saline, I promised her that if I was crazy enough to ever try a full Ironman, I'd hire a coach and train hard enough to finish the race and remain on my own two feet. Within a month I'd decided I was just that crazy.

Late in the fall of 2017, I hired coach Steve Brandes who started prescribing my daily training sessions. We worked around hospital, travel, and family commitments to build the endurance and power needed to withstand 12-14 hours of racing. I started training that winter with 30 minutes a day four to five days a week, and gradually expanded both time and intensity. By the summer of 2018, I was up every weekday morning at 4:30 a.m. to train for an hour and had one long run and one long ride each weekend. In August I raced in another half-distance Ironman 70.3 and finished almost an hour and a half faster than I'd finished the race in Raleigh—and I was well enough to drive myself home.

The summer stretched on and so did the workouts, with weekend sessions reaching at their longest over five hours of cycling one day and three hours of running the next. For months, my incredibly supportive family built our weekends around my training, and I finished nearly every training session Steve prescribed to the letter.

Finally, the day came, and October 14 wound up being ridiculously cold for Kentucky in early fall. The thermometer registered a balmy 48 degrees as a cold rain fell on the starting line, and I jumped into the Ohio river just after 9 a.m. for a current-shortened swim. It was just as cold a short while later when I finished the swim, waved to my wife and kids in the transition zone, and hopped on my bike to start the 112-mile journey around northwest Kentucky.

It was at this point that I seriously began to wonder whether I'd actually be able to finish the race. Having been burned by the heat in Raleigh the summer before, I'd trained in the hottest summer heat North Carolina had to offer and was ready to sweat. I was not, however, ready to shiver, and for the first 90 minutes of cycling I shivered in ways I didn't realize were physically possible. With the rain still falling and the thermometer stalled at 50 degrees, my clothes were soaked through within minutes. My face shook, my fingers shook, my arms shook, and every time I steered the bicycle down a hill, my entire body shook so hard I had a difficult time controlling the bike's handlebars. I honestly believed that if I kept going, I'd sooner or later lose control of the bike speeding down a hill and crash. Not willing to risk dying somewhere on a highway outside of La Grange, I knew there was no way I could finish the race without catching some kind of break.

It came just after mile 26 when I stopped at a high school with an aide station. A volunteer grabbed my bike, pulled me off, and directed my shuddering frame through the school's front doors. I walked into the lobby and found 50 other triathletes all shaking from the same hypothermia as me, caused by a combination of cold wind, cold rain, and a total lack of waterproof clothing. A second volunteer sent me into the men's restroom under the hot hand-dryer vents, which began to rewarm me instantaneously. It took 20 minutes for the shaking to subside, after which I found a seat in the makeshift field hospital.

The high school field hospital marked the beginning of the bike course's major loop, and it would be a solid two hours of cycling before I'd be able to get back to it. I knew there was no way I could make it two hours without a return of the uncontrollable shaking. I couldn't risk crashing, but I couldn't give up. I'd spent hundreds of hours in the pool, on my bike trainer, and pounding the pavement in my Nikes over the last year training for that day. I had a crew of friends and family rooting for me at home and watching my progress on the Ironman race app, which at that moment said only that I had gone "off course." And somewhere out on the race course, my wife and kids—who had sacrificed just as much as I had to make this day a possibility—were shivering themselves, waiting to root me on and cheer as I crossed the finish line that night. I desperately needed some kind of break. It turned out to be Mylar.

Most people only experience Mylar in shiny balloon form. Little known to those outside medicine is that Mylar is also an incredibly cheap but incredibly useful material for treating hypothermia, constructed of a very thin, very light plastic sheet coated with a metallized film. Like generations of endurance athletes before me, I had been wrapped in a Mylar blanket as soon as I entered the school and its reflective coating had helped warm me up from the inside out by preventing heat from escaping my body. Mylar blankets make for a terrific field hospital tool, but aren't particularly practical for riding a bicycle unless you're going for the caped crusader look. That didn't stop the volunteer at my table, though, who said, "Well why don't we just totally wrap you in it mummy-style?" Why not indeed.

She left for a moment and returned with more Mylar, a pair of scissors, and some tape. I unzipped my race jersey, and we wrapped the Mylar completely around my skin from chin to belly button, over each shoulder, and down each arm to my fingers. She then taped up all the seams and I zipped back up my jersey. I looked like the Tin Man and sounded like Jiffy Pop every time I moved, but it worked. Once I hit the course again, I found I could ride the downhills without shivering—my face, fingers, and feet were numb, but my core was warm and that's all that mattered.

As you'd expect, the rest of the race brought a few more obstacles. Around mile 80, I face-planted outside of an aide station when my bike ran over a Gatorade bottle. Mercifully, I was going close to zero MPH, and with the small laceration on my leg just as numb as the rest of me, it didn't take much extra resolve to push on. Seven hours after leaving the transition zone to start the bike leg, I finally rolled back into the transition zone, high-fived my kids again, and hit the run course.

With a little more luck, a lot of perseverance, and more Mylar than the Macy's Thanksgiving Day parade, I ultimately finished the race's final leg (the marathon) another four and a half hours later. I crossed the finish line at 4th Street Live in Downtown Louisville at 9:39 p.m., and was so deliriously overcome with emotion that I didn't even hear the iconic "Chris DeRienzo - You Are an Ironman!" announcer's call until a friend sent me the video she'd recorded live on her phone. It didn't matter—I hadn't given up, I'd stayed in the race long enough to catch a break, crossed the finish line on my own two feet, and walked back to the hotel with my wife and barely awake kids to celebrate.

In 10 years of practice, I've had many professional experiences where—just like in Ironman—the chips have been down and I thought we were out of options, but wasn't ready to give up. In rare circumstances, there truly has been no other viable option but to fold my cards, and I could be justly faulted in retrospect for enduring too long on a hopeless, even foolish, and unproductive mission. However, I've found the number of those circumstances to be vanishingly small compared to the number of times that continuing to persevere in medicine, especially NICU medicine, pays off. Stay in the game long enough and something almost always happens—something unexpected and rarely predict-able, like one final bolus of epinephrine, a last look at an echocardiogram, or magic Mylar.

I remember working with a partner one night on a baby who desperately needed an umbilical catheter. We had no other option to secure intravenous access, and spent hour after hour trying to thread a line of any kind into any one of the infant's three umbilical vessels. We tried cutting the cord sideways, we tried cutting it long-ways, and we tried cutting it a third time right down the middle. We used large lines and small lines, Iris forceps and Adson forceps, Kelly clamps and needle drivers. We tried every trick in every book we'd ever read, moving the infant's legs back and forth under the sterile drapes and gently directing the umbilical line up and down, left and right, back and forth, sideways and spiral-ways. No matter what we tried, the line simply wouldn't thread past the bend where an infants' umbilical vessels exit the superficial tissues and enter the deep, wide channels that lead into the heart. As we neared the end of our third hour under the bright warmer bed lights, we were both prepared to throw in the towel.

Soaked in sweat, our brows having been repeated-ly wiped by the infant's nurse and respiratory therapist and unclear what our next option would be, I remember saying I'd give it exactly one last try. I distinctly recall looking up to the ceiling over my glasses and mask and saying a Hail Mary. I'm not a deeply religious person, but at that point I thought it couldn't possibly hurt. For reasons I can't explain, I then had an idea and bent a pair of Iris forceps in half so they looked like wings. My partner looked at me wide-eyed over her face shield, but quickly caught on to where I was going. She grabbed two needle-drivers and held up what was left of the baby's umbilical cord while I re-flushed the umbilical line. With my left hand, I ever so gently teased open the lumen of what I thought could be the umbilical vein with the backwards-bent Irises, and with my right hand, I twisted the catheter through the tiny opening in one smooth pass. We stared at each other in amazement as the line slipped effortlessly through the infant's umbilical vein so deep it nearly reached the heart, as if all along it was just waiting—quite literally—for a wing and a prayer. When I pulled back on the plunger, I've never been so happy to see free-flowing blood filling a syringe. I've also never secured a tighter umbilical line in my career.

On another night, I remember working with a tremendously talented pediatric surgeon. We had a very small, very premature infant who was a few weeks old and whose umbilical lines had long since been removed. After about a week, if a baby still needs central intravenous access, the NICU team generally replaces his umbilical lines with something called a peripherally inserted central venous catheter (PICC). This infant indeed had a PICC line, but he had come down with a severe infection, which meant the line had to be removed. No one could find anywhere else to place another PICC or even just a regular IV, and he was going to need many weeks of intravenous antimicrobial medication to clear the infection and have a chance at survival.

Under these circumstances, pediatric surgeons generally have one of two options. Using a cut-down procedure like the one I described for ECMO, they can place a central intravenous line either into the jugular vein in the neck or into a similarly large vessel in the groin called the femoral vein. In order to perform either of these procedures, though, an infant has to be big enough for a physician to actually fit a catheter into one of these vessels. This infant wasn't even close, weighing in at just over a pound and with a femoral vein about the same size as a strand of angel hair pasta.

At that point, the surgeon and I looked at each other and wondered if there was any chance the same kind of cut-down procedure would be able to provide access to the long-ago closed off umbilical vessels. Even in adults, these vessels are never completely gone, slowly turning into fibrous bands of tissue that stay with us for the remainder of our lives. Given that this baby was still only a couple of weeks old—and that we quite literally had nothing else we could try—the surgeon agreed to try the umbilical cut-down. He would, however, need to perform the procedure at the baby's bedside and—given the nature of the case and without a pediatric surgery fellow available to help him—I had to agree to scrub in with him.

I am not a surgeon and hadn't scrubbed into a surgery since medical school, but I wasn't going to be the one remaining obstacle between this baby and his "never give up" option so in I scrubbed. We explained the procedure to the infant's parents, noting while the surgery itself was not inherently any riskier than any other kind of surgical cut-down, neither of us had ever actually tried this particular approach before. Nonetheless, it was the only option we had left. The parents quickly consented and the team went to work setting up an operating theatre right there in the middle of the NICU.

After an appropriate surgical timeout—the only time either of us have or likely will perform a timeout for an umbilical cut-down peripherally inserted central venous catheter placement procedure—we gave pain medicine and a paralytic, and I assisted the surgeon as he made a very small incision just below the baby's belly button. Sure enough, within half a centimeter or so of gentle blunt dissection, there was a blood vessel staring us both right in the face. We had no idea if it was an artery or a vein, but when the surgeon secured it and deftly passed the smallest PICC line the hospital carried into its lumen, we somehow found flowing venous blood.

I will never forget the look in the pediatric surgeon's dark eyes as they peered up through his magnifying glasses at me. His pupils looked like saucers through his special binocular loupes as he stood in disbelief and said, "I have no idea where this line is, and no idea where it's going, but we have blood return and we may have just saved this baby's life." He secured the line, sutured the skin closed, and we immediately began flushing the tiny line with intravenous fluids so it wouldn't clot. A portable radiograph showed that—amazingly—the infant's umbilical vein hadn't completely closed off and we had somehow found a way to curlicue the tiny catheter into its lumen and re-cannulate a small portion of the vessel. That implausible line—a literal life-line for that incredibly sick baby—wound up lasting for weeks, providing the access needed to give the baby enough antimicrobial medication to beat the infection. To this day, I wish I had saved that curlicue x-ray—I'd have it framed as one of the best radiographic examples of never giving up I will ever encounter.

That said, the greatest living example of "never give up" I've been fortunate enough to meet is a little girl named Alyssa. You wouldn't know it looking at the rambunctious preschooler she is today, but when she was born, Alyssa was the smallest human being that I and most of the Mission Hospital NICU team in Asheville, North Carolina, had ever seen. Her story has been shared with the world through her mother Haley's advocacy, Asheville's local country radio station 99.9 KISS FM, and a YouTube video titled "All God's Grace in One Tiny Face—Alyssa's journey."[5] I first met her, however, when she was much, much smaller.

It was the spring of 2015, and I was in my second year as an attending neonatologist serving the Mission Hospital Level III NICU. I'd come into the hospital one May morning for another day on-service on the NICU's Green Team. Just as in fellowship, I walked into the team room in my sea-green scrubs with caffeination in hand and took my seat at the sign-out table. From what I can remember, it was a fairly busy service, and the night-shift team started by talking about the significant overnight events on the babies we already knew. They breezed through the list, and I jotted down a few notes to follow up on after the handoff was complete.

Then they began signing out the new admissions, babies who had arrived to the unit since the day team had left around 5 p.m. the day before. The overnight doctor gave the Blue Team a few of the new babies, then he turned and stared at me with a look on his face that hovered between incredulous and amazed. He said that in the NICU's "D pod," back by the large-pane glass windows lit each morning by sunrise streaming over the Blue Ridge Mountains, he'd admitted one of the tiniest preemies he'd ever seen. She was just over 26 weeks gestation and weighed only 360 grams. I nearly fell out of my chair. I definitely spilled my coffee.

In the universe of preemies, the World Health Organization (WHO) uses a few categories to distinguish the small from the very small from the extremely small. The first WHO category is "low birthweight" or LBW,

---

which applies to any baby born weighing less than 2,500 grams or about 5 1/2 pounds. My brother, born a few weeks early and less than 5 pounds at birth, was characterized as LBW. The next category is VLBW, which stands for "very low birthweight" and includes infants born weighing less than 1,500 grams or a little over 3 pounds. Most 30-weekers and below fall into the VLBW category. "Extremely low birthweight" or ELBW is the most recently added WHO category and counts among its members infants born weighing less than 1,000 grams, or just over 2 pounds. ELBWs are generally around 28 weeks gestation or less, and as a category have a wide distribution of chances for survival and likelihood of experiencing any one of prematurity's most challenging morbidities.

WHO doesn't even have a category for infants like Alyssa who weigh less than 500 grams at birth. In fact, many NICU research studies and the Agency for Healthcare Research and Quality's[6] "Neonatal Mortality Rate" metric itself specifically exclude infants who weigh less than 500 grams at birth given the incredibly high variability in their survival rate.

Despite her infinitesimal size, Alyssa had one big thing going for her physiologically—her age. A weight of 360 grams would be small for even a 22-week fetus still growing inside her mother. That meant Alyssa had to be growth-restricted, so her body was much smaller than expected for her gestational age but likely just as mature as the body of a normally sized 26-weeker. Most 26-weekers are born weighing close to 800 grams and their chances of survival are much higher than infants born between 22 and 23 weeks in part because their

---

6   https://www.qualityindicators.ahrq.gov/.../NQI_02_Neonatal_Mortality_Rate.pdf

brains, lungs, and other organs have had three more weeks to mature before being exposed to the harsh realities of the world outside the womb. Three weeks may not seem like much, but remember every day a fetus spends inside her mother is more important and involves more rapid change than she will ever experience again. Alyssa was an 800-gram 26-weeker trapped in a 360-gram body, and we had to find a way to keep her alive and well long enough to just start growing.

Within days, Alyssa was both incredibly small and incredibly sick. On her third night, she came very close to dying from a pulmonary hemorrhage, and I sat with her parents Haley and Charles in our small NICU family room and talked through all of the possible ups and downs to come. Incredibly, by morning it was clear that she had survived the hemorrhage, though she still wouldn't be stable enough for her mother to hold her until she was 10 days old. Even then, it took a gaggle of people to make sure her breathing tube, countless sensors, and multitude of intravenous drips all stayed perfectly secure.

For four and a half months, Haley said the whole family "ran on caffeine and faith." She wasn't kidding. Premature infants are, unsurprisingly, also born with premature brains and premature brains often forget to breathe. While babies are growing inside their mothers, they really have no need to breathe—their lungs aren't exchanging oxygen and carbon dioxide. Instead, the placenta takes care of that job in addition to providing all the nutrients needed to slowly transform sperm and egg into a fully grown human infant. As a result, the "breathing center" in a baby's brain may not fully mature until closer to 34-36 weeks and sometimes even longer, which leaves 26-week preemies like Alyssa vulnerable to episodes of apnea.

In the 1970s, scientists discovered that chemicals called "methylxanthines" seemed to reduce or even eliminate these apneic episodes in premature infants. Within a few years of the research being published, drugs like aminophylline and theophylline became mainstays in NICUs all over the world. Over the last two decades, though, caffeine—which is also a methylxanthine—has become the drug of choice. It's much easier to give (see Dr. Abraham Verghese's fantastic book *Cutting for Stone* for a fictional but somewhat realistic example) and you have to give an awful lot of it to get any toxic side effects like fast heart rate or hyperactivity. By the time Alyssa was born in 2015, the standard loading dose of caffeine for apnea of prematurity was in the range of 20 milligrams per kilogram of an infant's bodyweight and some European neonatologists were studying doses as high as 40 milligrams per kilogram.

While premature infants metabolize caffeine much differently than adults, it's worth doing a little math to put this dose in perspective. The website CaffeineInformer.com tells me an average Grande Starbucks regular coffee contains around 300 milligrams of caffeine. This means a 70-kilogram man like me would need to drink nearly 10 Grandes in a row (or a full gallon plus a quart) to get the same caffeine load as a premature infant in the high-dose arm of the European NICU study. Give me that much coffee in one shot and I'd quickly progress from wide-awake, to hyperactive, to levitating, to dead. But for Alyssa it was a salvation, a drug that helped keep her breathing for many, many weeks until her brain could take over on its own.

For four and a half months, she caffeinated, learned to breathe, and learned to eat all while battling her premature lungs, problems with her heart, multiple bouts of infection, and more. Through it all, she typified Helena's words from Shakespeare's *A Midsummer Night's Dream*: "And though she be but little, she is fierce." She was remarkably little at first but remarkably strong, and proved to be just as fierce as the weeks passed and she grew and grew. I remember being on-call one night in mid-October when Alyssa and her parents were in the NICU's transition rooms, and being amazed that she was then almost the size of a full-term newborn. But for the tiny oxygen cannula around her nose, it would have been hard to tell from holding her that she had entered the NICU nearly five months earlier and around eight times smaller than when she finally got to go home.

Once Alyssa was discharged from the NICU, her strength only continued to grow. Within months, she weaned off the flicker of oxygen that she still had needed when she left the NICU. By the time I saw her in the NICU follow-up clinic the following year, she was crawling all over the floor with the physical therapist and gumming Gerber baby foods. We discharged Alyssa from our follow-up clinic at the age of 2, having fully caught up on all her developmental skills. A remarkable achievement for any 26-weeker, and practically unthinkable for one born the same size as a soda can.

In the spring of 2017, I was lucky to get to spend some time with Haley, Charles, and Alyssa at Asheville's March for Babies, an event sponsored by the March of Dimes. The March of Dimes is a non-profit organization that—having reached its goal of effectively ridding the world of polio—turned its attention to ensuring all babies (and their moms) have a healthy start in life. March of Dimes funding supports prematurity research at some of America's largest academic medical centers, and much of that funding comes from teams who raise money walking in Marches for Babies all over the country. At the Asheville March that day, Alyssa was the star of the show, a toddling 2-year old with beaming parents and a story that inspires in its sheer impossibility. She's now in preschool, and the world continues to make way for a tiny legend who knows where she's going.

More than anything else, I believe the spirit of healthcare is kindled by never giving up even in the face of extreme adversity. Yes, there are times the house will ultimately win, and yes, this approach to practicing medicine (and to life, for that matter) is bound to ultimately be wrought with examples of inevitable failures. Yet I remain convinced it's better than any other alternative, and stories like Alyssa's reinforce this belief for me every single day.

Alyssa's parents call her their hero. She is (and they are) much more than that. Perseverance may have made me become an Ironman, and Churchill's resolve may have sewn the sinews of peace amidst an iron curtain, but nothing I've read or experienced comes close to embodying the spirit of "never give up" more than Alyssa Summey. She is the "never give up" Iron Preemie, and would make even Snoopy proud.

Epilogue

"Life's like a movie,
Write you own ending,
Keep believing, keep pretending
We've done just what we've set out to do,
Thanks to the lovers,
The dreamers,
And you."

–Kermit the Frog: *The Muppet Movie*

It's been my sincerest hope to use this book as a vehicle to share with you a glimpse into the real world of practicing medicine. My real world of practicing medicine. One with fantastically fast-paced progress paired with the slow, intense struggle through uncertainty and doubt. Moments of stratospheric yet evanescent triumphs coupled with the inevitable haymakers, mistakes, and failures that piled up one upon the other can pave the road into burnout. Patients who will never forget their doctor and those whom their doctor will never forget. Life and death, sometimes spaced by decades and other times spaced by mere seconds.

Every doctor has his or her own stories and these have been mine. They of course aren't only mine, as I've shared a role in shaping them with patients, parents, families, colleagues, children, mentors, and friends, most of whom have remained nameless or have been altered in some small but meaningful way to protect their personal anonymity. Were they, however, to tell you the same stories, I'd not only expect a few interesting twists but imagine they would share views that often align with but occasionally diverge from my own.

And that's OK. Each of us lives our own unique life, creating our own personal narrative along the way to both explain the experiences of our day-to-day existence and connect the totality of those experiences to some larger arc of history. I've chosen to share these stories and their very personal connections to my own life, in hopes that they will help you better see the humanity in the humans surrounding you who are engaged in the delivery of healthcare. Some of my stories have been intended to make you laugh, others to make you cry, and others to make you scratch your head in either amazement or confusion. Whether I've succeeded or failed in doing so, time will tell.

In Chapter 5, I shared one of my favorite quotes from the Venerable Mother Catherine McAuley on striving to be good today but better tomorrow. The pursuit of continuous improvement is one of my life's core principles, and while Sister McAuley's words express it best, it's the words of President Theodore Roosevelt that best capture how to live it.

Teddy Roosevelt is one of my favorite historical figures, and in 1908 he wrote in a letter to the journalist Lincoln Steffans defending his approach to leadership that (and I'm paraphrasing here): "Real progress is won by people who take the next step, not those who theorize about the 200th." It's the second of two of my favorite quotes that I couldn't work into one of this book's chapter titles. Despite the colossal influence of trusts like Standard Oil, Roosevelt lived this "take the next step" approach to driving progress. In doing so, he managed to band together coalitions of progressive Republicans and Democrats to drive real progress in America on everything from the quality and safety of the nation's meat supply to campaign finance reform. While each victory was imperfect, all moved the health of the nation purposefully forward both economically and socially. Teddy Roosevelt sought to make America better by focusing his energies on driving us to take the next step.

My closest family and friends can testify that I've never been a particularly open person. While what you see is what you get in terms of honesty and transparency, I usually hold the most personal aspects of my life, my stories, and how I think and feel about them fairly close to my chest. That said, I'm deeply passionate about healthcare and about sharing the incredible humanity I've seen ingrained in the practice of medicine. The human experience is best shared through storytelling—I've always enjoyed writing, and have wanted to share these stories with the world for a long time. Thus, for the last two years, I've imagined a small, mustachioed, pistol-carrying and hyperkinetic Theodore Roosevelt perched on my shoulder spurring me to keep writing this book. *Tiny Medicine* is where I needed to go, so I pointed my feet in its general direction and took the next step.

More than anything else, I hope *Tiny Medicine* leaves you with a sense of wonder about medicine and the human experience of practicing it as a physician. The stories that make up my life as a doctor make me feel lucky to be an American physician in the early 21st century.

I am fortunate to have spent the last 10 years serving thousands of patients both in practice and in leadership. I am fortunate to be working at a time when the American healthcare system acknowledges the inevitability of human error and is firmly committed to continuously improving until we can prevent any error from reaching a patient and causing harm. Finally, I'm incredibly lucky to have been given the time, energy, and ability to write this book, which was as much catharsis and celebration for me as (hopefully) entertainment for you. And I am eternally grateful that you have read it.

My favorite television show of all time is *The West Wing*. It was about life in the fictional administration of President Jed Bartlet, and aired for seven seasons on NBC in the early 2000s. In an episode titled "Noël" during the second (and by far best) season, a character named Josh is in the midst of a burnout-like downward spiral as a result of post-traumatic stress from an event earlier in the season. By the end of the hour-long episode, he's just begun to acknowledge the depth of his suffering and recognize how close he's come to finding the bottom of his own well. He walks out of the White House conference room in which he's spent his entire Christmas Eve with two counselors from the American Trauma Victims Association coming to terms with his circumstances, when he runs into his boss Leo McGarry. He asks Leo why he's still there waiting for him on Christmas Eve, and Leo tells Josh the following story:

"This guy's walking down the street when he falls in a hole. The walls are so steep he can't get out. A doctor passes by and the guy shouts up, 'Hey you. Can you help me out?' The doctor writes a prescription, throws it down in the hole, and moves on. Then a priest comes along and the guy shouts up, 'Father, I'm down in this hole. Can you help me out?' The priest writes out a prayer, throws it down in the hole, and moves on. Then a friend walks by, 'Hey, Joe, it's me. Can you help me out?' And the friend jumps in the hole. Our guy says, 'Are you stupid? Now we're both down here.' The friend says, 'Yeah, but I've been down here before and I know the way out.'"

Now that we have shared these deeply personal stories, you too can consider yourself a friend in the hole. You know what it feels like for a doctor to reach the peaks of professional joy, to plumb to the bottoms of his professional valleys, and to live every day in the space in between. You've been there with me and made it through to the end, and now you too know the way out. It's no secret—healthcare is about humans, even when the humans are as small as a can of soda.

In closing, the next time you're in the kitchen fixing yourself a sandwich, a fruit salad with grapes, and a soda with a straw in the can, I hope that you'll pause for just a moment and think about the 15 million premature infants born worldwide each year. Think about how impossibly small they really are and the impossibly long odds so many of them face to survive. Think about how incredible it is to live at a time when science and medicine allows us to save babies born 12 times smaller than they should be and more than four months too soon. Think about their families, spending hour after hour next to their isolettes, celebrating each day and worrying each night and never giving up until there is truly no choice but to do otherwise.

Perhaps most importantly, stop and think about the people. Think about the doctors, nurses, students, trainees, respiratory therapists, pharmacists, aides, clerks, and countless other team members who spend their entire professional lives in service of children and their parents. Think about the inevitable peaks and valleys they have walked through learning and living their professions, and about the impossibility of preventing the bleeding they see and experience at work from seeping into their lives at home. Make sure to pray for the ones who are suffering at the moment in their career when they tap the bottom of their well, and if you know who they are and they are among your closest friends, just take the next step, jump into the well with them. You know the way out and can help them turn the light back on.

And when you do, remember that medicine is now, and always will be, a uniquely human endeavor.

Acknowledgments

I owe countless debts of gratitude for this book and my life in medicine. First and foremost, I am the luckiest, most grateful husband and father on planet earth. It takes superhuman patience and understanding to spend a lifetime with me. Fortunately for me, I married a superhuman and we have three superhuman children who find new ways to scare me witless, make me smile, make me laugh, and make me profoundly proud on a daily basis.

To Drs. Ronald Goldberg, David Tanaka, Margarita Bidegain, Susan Izatt, C. Michael Cotten, P. Brian Smith, Jeffrey Ferranti, and the rest of the Duke Neonatology faculty—you believed in me even when I didn't believe in myself, and for that, words cannot express my thanks. To Dr. Ron Paulus, thank you for seeing a kid who reminded you a little of yourself, for investing in me, for being patient and willing to both weather and coach me through the inevitable failures that come with youth and inexperience, and for giving me way more chances to prove myself than I deserved. To Drs. Mary-Ellen Taplin, Deb Squire, Karen Frush, Tom Owens, John Ball, and Jill Hoggard-Green—you saw something in me I didn't know was there, invested your time to mentor, direct, and shape a young leader with promise, and for that I can never fully express my gratitude.

To my in-laws Ronnie and Pat Fowlkes, you welcomed me into your family with open arms despite my Yankee upbringing, made me feel at home, and shower love upon my children as frequently and as deeply as I do. To Liz Boehm, Aurora Aguilar, Bridget Duffy, Nate Klemp, R.J. Salus, Scott Becker, and all the friends and colleagues who've helped shape this book and prodded me onward past roadblock after roadblock, thank you for pushing me over the finish line. To Ann Young, thank you for being able to see things I'd simply have no other way to see, and for your incredible generosity with your time, your energy, and your red editorial ink. To Eric Langshur, for taking a flyer on supporting me in writing this book and for authoring a foreword better than I could possibly have imagined.

To my team at Mission Health, including Chris Shelton, Robert Whiteside, Stephanie Baron, Victor McHenry, Kristin Patton, and Micah Krempasky. I have been tremendously fortunate to work with such a talented, dedicated, and energetic group. Thank-you for just being who you are – keep going. To Dr. Shannon Dowler, while I am certain I'll never be able to rap with your particular combination of skill and panache, I hope to be able to lead with your singular sense of purpose, your commitment to inalienable core values, and your seemingly endless drive. To Linda Hummel, the only other recipient of the Dr. Paulus "Unvarnished Praise Award," we've proved how a millennial and a boomer can move mountains together and it's been the privilege of my career to be your partner. To Melanie Hensley, without your constant energy, strength, and compassion for these past five years, I'd have never eaten, slept, or seen my family—thank you for finding ways to make everything work, no matter how frequently I find new and interesting ways to mess it up.

To the soon-to-be Dr. Stephen Kircher and to Haley, Charles, and Alyssa Summey, thank you for your willingness to contribute to this story and for all that you've done past and present to make me a better doctor and a better person. To the countless Duke pediatric and NICU nurses and nurse practitioners, thank you for raising me up as a medical student and a young doctor, weaning me from academics, teaching me to believe in myself, and sending me on my way. To the thousands of nurses and other team members across Mission Health I've been privileged to work with for the last five years as a partner, thank you for your never-ending dedication to serving our people and our communities. To Ms. Bell and Mrs. Badavas—thank you for driving both an appreciation for commas and fanatically correct grammar into my high-school-aged brain. And of course, to my editor, publisher, and literary sensei Kevin Murphy—we believed in each other in our own respective early days, and I'm proud of where we've both come together.

Finally, to my parents for molding me into the person I am—continuously curious, driven to get better every day, genetically incapable of accepting the answer "just because," and only able to accept defeat when someone is smarter, faster, or stronger, but never just because I didn't work hard enough. As a father of three children of my own, I am only now realizing how hard this parenting thing is to do so well. Know that you did, and a thousand lifetimes wouldn't be long enough to be able to repay the debt.

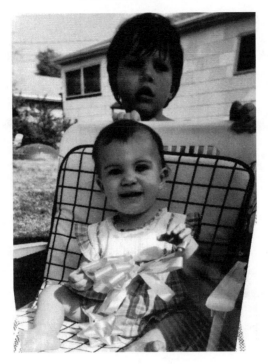

With my sister and the infamous bush in the backyard of our house in Commack, NY. Note the look of extreme concern on my face ... those bows could be dangerous. (1985)

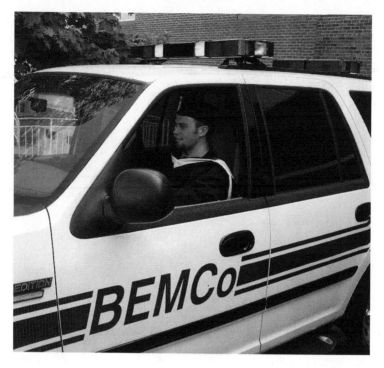

Driving the Brandeis Emergency Medical Corps Supervisor Truck after college graduation, and wondering why I ever thought goatees were "in." (2003)

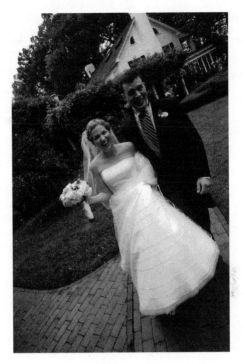

With Melody on our wedding day. It had poured rain the night before and the pair of pearl-colored heels she bought sank in the wet grass, so if you look closely enough you can just make out the tip of the J. Crew sandals she wound up having to wear instead. (2006)

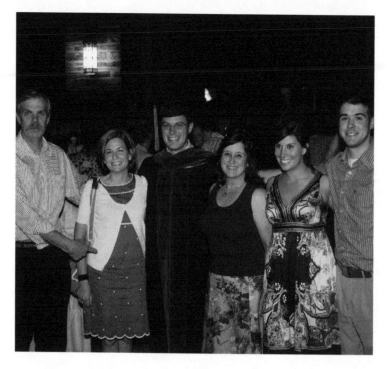

The newly-christened Dr. Chris DeRienzo, at my medical school graduation hooding ceremony with (left-to-right) my Dad, Melody, my Mom, my sister Lauren and my brother Michael. Melody was pregnant with our first baby, and my father (note where he's pointing) wanted to ensure she would eventually know she made it into the picture too. (2008)

Schedule for DeRienzo, Christopher 8-25 to 9-21, 2008   Yearly clinic summary   Weekends

6/26-7/27 (7/7)	7/28-8/24 (8/11)	8/25-9/21 (9/8)	9/22-10/19 (10/6)	10/20-11/16 (11/3)	11/17-12/21 (12/1)	12/22-12/27 (12/25)	12/28-1/2 (12/31)	1/3-2/1 (1/19)	2/2-3/1 (2/16)	3/2-3/29 (3/16)	3/30-5/3 (4/13)	5/4-5/31 (5/18)	6/1-6/30 (6/15)
SDC	DRH	HarrisInt2	Vac 10/6-10/12 Cards	KatzInt1	SDC	HarrisInt1	Vac	Newborn	FTN	NICUInt	DavInt2	ED | Vac	HowInt1

Su	Mo	Tu	We	Th	Fr	Sa
17 August	18 Mo	19 Tu	20 We	21 Th	22 Fr	23 Sa
DRH	DRH RR ↓	DRH	DRH	DRH	DRH	DRH DRHSr Short (
24 Su	25 Mo	26 Tu	27 We	28 Th	29 Fr	30 Sa
DRH	HarrisInt2 RR ↑	HarrisInt2	HarrisInt2 H-D WardInt (	HarrisInt2	HarrisInt2	HarrisInt2 Day off ↓
31 Su	1 Labor day	2 Tu	3 We	4 Th	5 Fr	6 Sa
HarrisInt2 H-D WardInt (	HarrisInt2	HarrisInt2 RR ↓	HarrisInt2	HarrisInt2 H-D WardInt (	HarrisInt2	HarrisInt2
7 September	8 Mo	9 Tu	10 We	11 Th	12 Fr	13 Sa
HarrisInt2 Day off ↓	HarrisInt2 H-D WardInt (	HarrisInt2	HarrisInt2	HarrisInt2 RR ↑	HarrisInt2 H-D WardInt (	HarrisInt2
14 Su	15 Mo	16 Tu	17 We	18 Th	19 Fr	20 Sa
HarrisInt2	HarrisInt2 RR ↑	HarrisInt2 H-D WardInt (	HarrisInt2	HarrisInt2 Day off ↓	HarrisInt2	HarrisInt2 H-D WardInt (
21 Su	22 Mo	23 Tu	24 We	25 Th	26 Fr	27 Sa
HarrisInt2	Cards RR ↑	Cards J Intern (	Cards Eye Center ↓	Cards SCOPE ↓ J Intern (	Cards Morning Report (	Cards

↑ = AM clinic   ↓ = PM clinic   (= On call

My actual intern year schedule, highlighting my first month on the "Harris" team when I met Stephen Kirchner. The "H-D WardInt" days with crescent moons were my call days/nights, and "RR" signaled mornings or afternoons where I went to clinic. You'll note the absence of a "golden weekend," intern-speak for getting both Saturday and Sunday off in a row. (2008–2009)

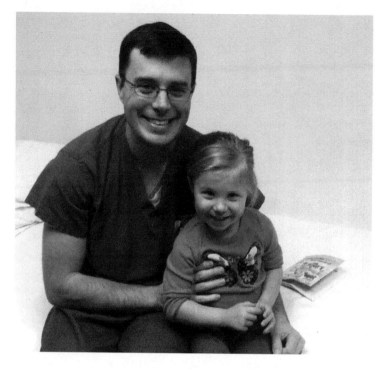

A surprise visit from our oldest during a call night in fellowship. Note the plywood-like call room bed we're sitting on and the Chick-Fil-A book that came with her kids' meal in the background. (2011)

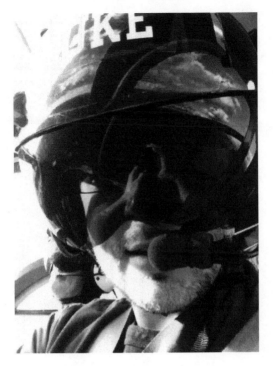

With the Duke LifeFlight helicopter crew en route to a call. On flights out when it was just the crew onboard, the former military pilots would occasionally hum "Ride of the Valkyries" over the headset speakers and really lean into the bank-turns ... I won't lie, it was awesome. (2011)

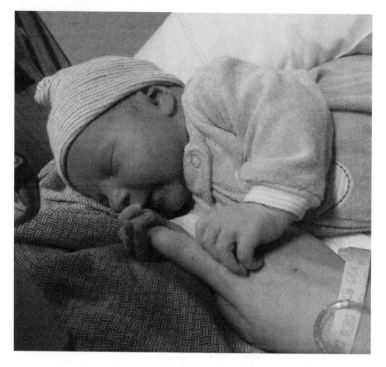

Our second child grasping her mother's finger soon after she was born. Look at how tiny her fingers seem compared to my wife's … and she weighed 9 pounds! (2012)

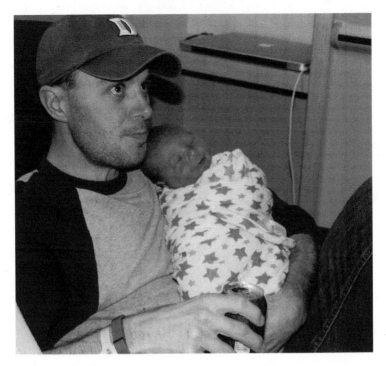

With my youngest watching the college football championship game barely 12 hours after he was born. I had a Coke. He opted for the breastmilk. (2014).

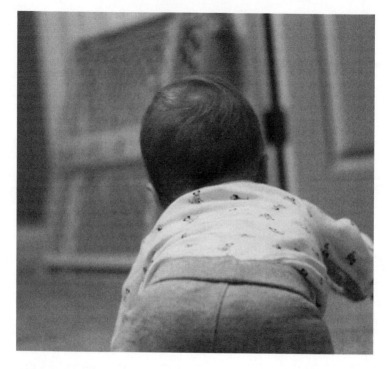

One small reach for man, one giant crawl for mankind ... (2014)

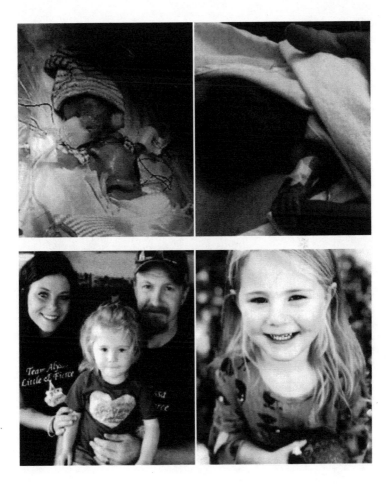

Clockwise from top left, Alyssa Summey: 1. In the NICU shortly after birth, 2. Holding a giant finger with such a tiny hand, 3.,With her parents Haley and Charles at the March of Dimes, and 4. As a rambunctious preschooler. I've never met, and will never meet, a more incredible preemie. (2015–2018)

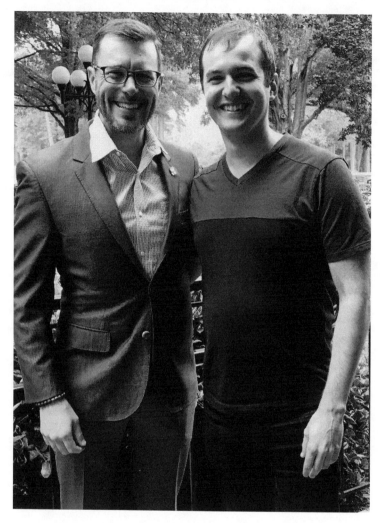

With Stephen Kirchner, now a third-year MD/PhD student, celebrating his total domination of Step 1 of the United States Medical Licensing Exam just over 10 years to the day after we first met on the pediatric oncology ward at Duke Hospital. (2018)

Learn more about Dr. Chris DeRienzo at

www.bigeyebooks.com